WEIGHT-LOSS
PSYCHOLOGY FOR WOMEN

Discover the Rapid Way for Female to Stop Emotional Eating & Burn Fat With Self-Hypnosis. Learn How to Lose Weight with Positive Affirmations and Guided Meditations

Keli Bay

Table of Contents

Introduction

Weight-loss psychology focuses on how people's thoughts, emotions, and behaviors contribute to their weight and body image. It also examines what can help them lose weight in beneficial ways.

A newfound study suggests that people who were more self-conscious about their food choices had lower body fat levels than those who were less concerned with what they ate. Another study found that obese dieters who spoke positively about themselves lost more weight than those who didn't voice such positivity.

You can feel healthier—A healthy body is a great feeling and a happy one. The truth is, once you take care of yourself by losing weight, you will be surprised at how much better you feel overall.

You can bring out the real you—Just like you see with children, watching yourself improve allows you to be a better role model than you were before. That is the beauty of weight loss. It improves your everyday life as well as your overall health.

Makes you feel better about yourself—There is no reason to feel ashamed of your body or what it looks like. Losing weight can bring out the best in all of us and help us appreciate our bodies more for all that they can do when cared for properly.

You can play a bigger role in your health—Women who lose weight have a better chance of living longer and controlling their blood pressure. Losing extra pounds also helps with the support of the organs, so that they can do their job optimally.

These pros can only be attained if you are ready to start your weight-loss journey. There are several ways tackled in this narrative about weight-loss psychology, as well as on how to effectively lose weight.

This feat is not an easy task because you have to be able to change your mindset and perspective to succeed. It's been proven that people who think they are fat when they are not, tend to have huge weight problems. The same is true for those who think they are as thin as a rail when they really aren't. It's a good idea to get your mindset in the right place. If you don't know your body type, go to the doctor and find out. You also have to understand that to lose weight, one has to know how to eliminate the unnecessary or superfluous interventions that are commonly suggested by the health industry. Oftentimes, the industry tries to exploit women especially on easy diet tips and tricks but we are here to educate on how to avoid falling into the industry's traps.

A lot of people believe that losing weight is impossible, especially when they're doing it for a long time already and have not seen any significant results yet.

However, you have to dig deep and learn more about weight-loss psychology to reactivate your slimming energy. In this way, you can prevent burnout from happening, and you will always be motivated to continue moving forward and not give up. It may be overwhelming, but once you have adequate knowledge, you will attain the results you have always dreamed of.

CHAPTER 1:

Find Your Natural Rhythm: Slow Down, Give Yourself the Right Time to Everything

The most important part of a weight-loss journey is time management. This doesn't mean setting a quick goal and achieving it as fast as possible. It's all about using time properly and understanding how long it takes to actually do something. We set ridiculous goals for ourselves in the hopes that we'll achieve something great, but what ends up happening is, as the end date approaches, we become overwhelmed and are set up for disappointment. We have to be realistic with our time goals and consider all factors when making different plans.

Practice Patience

Patience is hard to achieve. Anyone that wants to lose weight hopes that they can just jump on the scale after eating a salad and see the number drop by double digits. We have to accept before starting a weight-loss journey that this will never happen. We won't be able to just lose weight overnight.

Sometimes, patience is hard to have when exercising. Many people find themselves getting bored on treadmills or other machines that require a repetitive activity for minutes at a time. Use different exercise methods that you find fun or entertaining, such as a dance class or going on an interesting trail run. If the gym is your only option, use the boring moments on machines as a way to meditate. Clear your head, not thinking of how much weight you want to lose or what else you have to do to get there. Just practice counting or focusing on a quiet place you find peace in, such as a beach or a park. Visualize this to find a place for meditation. It'll take practice, but you'll soon find that you can zone out and work hard if you just focus.

There Is No Rush

Weight loss takes time; we can't emphasize that enough. Some diets and exercises will help you lose weight quicker than others, but overall, you're going to have to put in a lot of time to lose weight. Remember not to feel too rushed throughout this journey. You have to be strict and consistent to see results, but there's no point in forcing yourself into ridiculous time constraints. If you cause yourself anxiety over certain dates, you might feel the need to stress eat or go through dangerous dieting practices to get there.

Set Small Goals

Instead of looking at a wedding coming up in a couple of months as your goal for losing weight, instead, use that as a small milestone. Many of us get worried looking at the future, thinking of things coming up as the time limits for which we have to lose weight. Maybe it's March and you only have a couple of months until swimsuit season. Instead of going on a diet to lose thirty pounds in three months, use the beginning of summer as a small milestone in your journey. The aim, instead, to be healthier and more confident by the time summer comes, rather than giving yourself a ridiculous goal that you don't even know if you can achieve.

Don't Wait for Monday

Many people have an unhealthy perception of dieting when looking at certain periods. Maybe it's a Tuesday, and so they tell themselves that next Monday is going to be the date to start dieting. In preparation for that date, the same person might make sure to eat all the junk in their house to make sure temptation is removed. But then, by the time Monday comes, something else happens that delays it further.

Even worse, maybe it's Sunday night and you decide that since tomorrow is Monday, you're going to start your diet right now. But then, Tuesday comes, and the diet doesn't start, so you feel discouraged and you count that as just another time that you failed! Don't do this! Instead, set a starting point much further into the future. Find a date two weeks away, whether it's on a Monday, the first of the month, or just a random Wednesday. That way, you can prepare for the official diet-start date. This way, you can practice as the actual date approaches. For example, your New Year's resolution might be to lose weight. If that's the case, throughout December, you should practice incorporating workout routines a few times a week and experiment with healthy dinners. Then, when January comes around, you have more experience in dieting and are better prepared to start your journey than if you had only given yourself a few days to prep.

Something to Tend

Your weight is something to tend to. Think of it as a plant. You don't just plant a flower and walk away. The flower will grow, but if you don't go back and make sure to water it, the flower will die. Your journey is a flower. By purchasing this book, you've purchased the seeds. As you read these words, you're reading how to plant the seed and how to make sure that it stays alive. Once the flower blossoms, you'll have reached your weight-loss goal. Just like the flower, if you abandon your goals and don't tend to your weight-loss journey, you will fall off track and go back into your old lifestyle.

Lifestyle Change

Losing weight isn't just a reduction in numbers. It's a change in the entire way you live your life. Some people seem very thin and yet they might be able to eat whatever they want. These people give the illusion that if an overweight person becomes thin, they can then start to eat what they want. That's not how it works, however. Those thin people are just among the handful of individuals that were just born lucky! If you're overweight now, there's a good chance that it's part of your makeup, and weight fluctuations might just be something you have to learn how to manage.

This means you can't just cut out soda for a year, lose fifty pounds, and then start drinking soda again. The weight will come back if you don't manage your habits. That idea can be scary for some people. They might assume that they have to give up soda forever. That doesn't have to be the case. What has to change is just how much soda you can consume. If you drink a Coke a day, you might want to just give the Coke up, hoping you can go back to that behavior after you lose a certain amount of weight.

You have to accept that you can no longer drink a Coke every day if you want to keep up with your weight. Instead, maybe just have soda on weekends, or only when you're going out to eat. Find a way to incorporate the things you desperately love from your past life into your new healthy lifestyle.

Keeping the Weight Off

The part where many people really fall through with their goals is after they actually achieve them! Many people get to their desired weight, see that number, and think they no longer have to keep up with their diet plan. Then, the weight comes back, and the cycle of disappointment has to be lived all over again. Remember that once you reach your first goal, you should set another one. The second might not be as extreme. For example, maybe your first goal is to get down to 180 pounds. Once you do that, you have to come up with something new. That might be getting down to 170 pounds, or it could be something different, such as improving the muscle mass in a certain part of your body. Never stop setting goals. The level of difficulty can fluctuate. But to stay on track and keep the weight off, you have to continually encourage yourself to do better.

Change Things Up

Some people might find that after a year or two of dieting and exercising, they stop losing weight. This can be because their bodies are now used to healthy behavior. You probably won't ever lose as much weight in a diet as you do at the beginning. Those transformations can be invigorating, but remember that as you continue, it will become a little less drastic.

If you feel you've plateaued in your diet, you should consider changing things up. This might involve trying an entirely new diet, or it could be working out differently. Incorporating variety helps to ensure that you'll stick to your goals while also having fun!

Don't Revel in Regret

Once you reach your weight-loss goals, you might find yourself feeling regretful. Maybe you feel remorse over not doing it sooner. You might think to yourself about how if you had started exercising as a teen, it wouldn't be so hard to keep up with the weight now.

Don't blame your past self for what they didn't do. Instead, thank them for what they taught you. There is no going back in time. What happened, the decisions we made, and the weight we gained already occurred, and there's no reversing. Instead, we have to look at our past mistakes and use them as lessons. Remember that you wouldn't be the person you are right now if you hadn't experienced every single thing you did. The more you learn to love yourself, the better you'll be able to forgive the past "you" for all the things they did you wish they hadn't.

It Gets Easier

Always remember that it will get easier. You just have to get into a healthy lifestyle with good habits. The more practice you put into working out, and the more dedicated you are to your diet, the better you'll be able to manage your weight. The first day at the gym is going to be tough. You might be excited to start, but there also might be feelings of fear of judgment and anxiety that you might fail. Don't let anything discourage you from going back. Every time you walk through the doors of your gym or decide not to eat the candy in the workroom, remember that next time, it's going to get even easier.

The struggle doesn't end. Your legs will always be sore after an intense workout. You'll still sweat through your T-shirts, and you'll still crave all the sweets that caused the weight gain in the first place. Those difficulties don't just disappear. However, the more dedicated you are and the better focus you have on achieving your goals, the easier it gets every time.

Be Proud of Yourself

No matter where you are in your weight-loss journey, at any given time, you should be proud. The fact that you even want to change is something you should be proud of. It's not easy, and if it were, everyone would be thin and healthy. Even though you might want to blame yourself for being here in the first place, remember that positive reinforcement is the way you're going to be able to keep up with your goals.

Remember, It Is Up to You

You can use different tools, gym memberships, or workout gear to help encourage you to live a healthier lifestyle. At the end of the day, the only thing you can depend on is yourself.

CHAPTER 2:

Learn to Wait Without Anxiety

Diets cause stress and anxiety. We suffer stress when we force ourselves for some reason, and we suffer from anxiety when we afraid of failure. Stress and anxiety are two major reasons that we might discontinue a diet.

We feel anxious while dieting as we are afraid that we will be hungry all the time and will hence lose the pleasure of our food. In addition, we show anxiety symptoms when we believe that the diet will be unsuccessful. In conclusion, the diet is causing stress with a limited amount of food and anxiety because of the expected results. This combination guarantees failure!

Recently, anxiety-inducing headlines about weight loss and dieting have been popping up left and right. Outlet after outlet is reporting the latest in negative health news and the impact it has on self-esteem. We all know that worrying about our weight can be a vicious cycle, but that doesn't mean we should give up hope entirely.

Anxiety is like a never-ending cycle. When you have it, you look at yourself negatively, which makes it worse. You look at yourself more negatively, so you start to over-expect yourself, which makes it worse. That's how anxiety works—it loops back on itself. And this vicious cycle is what keeps people from reaching their goals.

But that doesn't mean we should give up hope entirely. There are activities you can execute to make your anxiety stop cycling and turn towards a path of success, such as having:

Self-Confidence

Self-confidence is the belief in ourselves that we can achieve the goals that we set. Somebody who has high self-confidence believes in himself and somebody who has low confidence believes that he will fail. High self-confidence is an important factor for a successful effort of weight loss. The failed attempts for slimming in people who have lost weight and regained pounds but who are on diets are negative factors for self-confidence. Someone who has repeatedly failed to lose weight doesn't believe in their power when they start a new diet.

Self-esteem is the impression that we have for ourselves. Self-esteem is high when we are satisfied with ourselves and low when we are disappointed. The failed attempts for slimming and frustration from the image of our body reduce our overall self-esteem. High self-esteem is associated with high confidence and contributes significantly to the success of weight loss.

Self-punishment and self-destruction are ways to relieve ourselves of our emotions. Usually, when we are disappointed about ourselves unconsciously or consciously, we want to punish ourselves.

The feelings of anger towards ourselves could easily lead us to destruction. Generally, feelings of anger should be defused or controlled. If those feelings are connected to a weight-loss program, we will have the opposite effect than expected.

Feelings of depression can also lead us to self-destruction. Freud's theory relates self-destruction to the instinct of death and claims that we lead ourselves to death during our life.

Reactance Theory

Reactance theory is a reactive behavior to the forbidden or the elimination of freedom. When desired behavior is banned, the person feels that freedom is challenged and tries to claim it in every way.

That person positively evaluates the forbidden behavior. For example, in a diet program, there are many forbidden foods. If the person feels restricted, he could easily express a different and opposite behavior than the proposed behavior. This theory explains various outbursts and irregularities during the diet program. At the same time, aggressive behavior could be developed towards ourselves and towards others who come into the same diet.

The Mistakes in Diets

The biggest mistake that people make in the diet is setting a very high goal. They have high expectations of themselves in a very short period of time. A goal to lose too many pounds seems unrealistic to everybody. In addition, a goal too high can cause stress and anxiety. It is much better if we set a goal to change the way of living than the weight loss. For sure, if we achieve the changing of our lifestyle, we will also achieve control of our weight.

Another huge mistake is the impression that we will be on a diet for a specific time and then return to our old habits. The "miracle diet" unfortunately does not exist. We come again to the conclusion that a permanent change of lifestyle will lead to permanent results in weight control.

As mentioned above, a serious mistake in any diet is a large calorie reduction. If we reduce dramatically the calorie intake, our body will experience extreme stress and it is completely normal for our body to react to this stress adversely. The larger and more abrupt the food reduction is, the higher the chance of failure and quitting the diet program.

The body tends to try to return to the balance that was required to maintain its former weight. For this reason, when we skip meals or when we reduce the amount of food, hunger symptoms become even more pronounced. In the long term, many failed diet attempts lead to weight gain rather than loss.

A psychological mistake in any diet is the connection of food intake with pleasure. People who diet set rules for themselves and they feel that they lose the pleasures in life. If we feel deprived in a diet program, we are bound to fail. The diet should give us positive feedback and be a behavior that we enjoy doing.

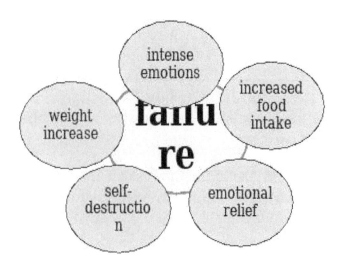

The Vicious Cycle Through Dieting

If the results of pressing diets are negative, we can be driven to feelings of frustration, anger, and self-destruction. That easily creates the vicious cycle of failed diets. Someone who is stressed when on a diet is 100% certain to fail. That failure will cause intense negative emotional feelings and self-destruction. The increase in food is the next step to relieve those feelings. The final result will be increased body weight and negative feelings.

To Succeed in Dieting

The first goal to lose weight should be a personal balance instead of a battle with the scales. Anyone who starts to lose weight should first be determined to:

- Change their life
- Be relaxed

The only certain way to achieve weight loss is by changing our lifestyle. We must apply the following behaviors to get results and lose weight:

- Application of daily exercise
- The understanding of satiation
- The disconnection of positive emotions with unhealthy foods
- The developments of confidence and self-control

Self-Observation

Observing ourselves before, during, and after a diet, any behavior will lead us to valuable conclusions. Sometimes we do not realize the emotional background of a behavior, like the thoughts that accompany behaviors or emotions. When we are conscious of our feelings and cause-connected behaviors, we can control them more easily. If we frequently repeat some eating habits, we connect eating with some behaviors and seek to repeat them continuously. For example, common behaviors are eating while we are watching TV, when we are using the PC, or when we are with friends. Most of the time eating includes unhealthy foods such as chips, crisps, popcorn, and soft drinks. We will explore later how we can use the technique of self-observation.

Anxiety can be a result of over-training, or the body adapting to an improved workout. People can overdo it on weightlifting, running, or cycling. The body begins to adapt to an improved workout due to stress hormones being pumped at a faster rate. The stress hormones cause the "fight or flight" response and the muscle fibers are pushed beyond what they're designed for. The end product is that you feel worn out and run down for no apparent reason. The problem is that if we feel "worn out," we are not motivated to push further in the workout. On top of that, anxiety tends to amplify the problems you have in life. This means that depressed people who worry about their weight will also feel more anxious about it. And anxiety tends to amplify other issues, like confidence issues, eating disorders, poor sleep habits, and poor self-image. Stress is a big factor in anxiety, and to relieve it you have to remove the stressor. Aside from the formerly mentioned steps, here are some of the simple steps to remove stressors:

First, take a "time out" from exercise so you can recover from over-training. Remove yourself from the weightlifting or cardiovascular exercise for up to two weeks while you focus on rebuilding your body's strength. The second is to find an exercise that doesn't cause anxiety, like walking or swimming.

Sleep Deprivation

There are vital hormones in the body that process information and release them into the brain. These hormones play a role in mood and can be affected by poor sleeping habits. In particular, REM sleep is when your body repairs itself, so it's a fantastic time to relax and unwind. If you don't get enough sleep, then anxiety levels will rise.

If you're having trouble getting sleep at night, try a holistic approach to things. Get more exercise throughout the day to relax in the evening. Mindfulness is also a great way to deal with anxiety and stress. You can learn how to meditate and "be in the moment." This will help your brain properly rest and unwind.

A lot of people are anti-medication, but if you really struggle with sleep issues and anxiety, it may be worth it for you. It's important to ensure you're always within the recommended dosage and consult with a physician.

Positive Thinking

Psychologists have found that positive thinking can be the best way to deal with anxiety. This is because it helps the mind process information without freaking out. If you want to wake up feeling relaxed and refreshed, then positive thinking is one of the most effective methods.

It's also important to not overdo things. Don't place too much burden on your shoulders to find the "right" way of life. If you feel like you're going to fail, then it's best to take a step back and consider a different approach.

Meditation

Meditation is an appropriate way to relax and relieve some stress. There are countless techniques and programs out there, but The Mindful Way to Heal is one of the most popular methods. It combines a lot of science with mindfulness.

If you want to try meditation then you need to embrace the process. It can be frustrating at first because there are no overnight results. But if you stick with it and give your mind time to unwind, then meditation can be one of the best ways to feel calm and stress-free. For beginners, try doing 20 minutes per day and slowly work towards an hour.

Stick With It

Remember that confidence is key in reaching your goals. Focus on all the good things about yourself. Keep your self-esteem in check by thinking about all the things you can do and the skills you have. Don't rely too heavily on other people, and don't worry about what others think of you.

You're the only one who can evaluate your life and decide if something needs to change or not. Be confident in yourself, stick with it, and know that there are many ways to deal with anxiety.

CHAPTER 3:

Discover the Powers of Distraction: Let Your Mind Run Free With Memories, Fantasies

Several studies have been conducted to find a link between distraction and weight loss. One study found that when participants were distracted while dieting, they ate less and shed weight more effectively than people who were not distracted. Another study also found that the level of distraction did not affect whether people lost weight or gained it.

The thing is the key to losing weight isn't about how you feel or what you do; it's all about calories in versus calories out. If you produce more energy than you consume, you will lose weight. It doesn't matter if you do it on purpose or by accident. The important thing to remember is that weight loss is not the result of your efforts. It's the result of a caloric imbalance.

A myriad of studies has been implemented to see if distraction affects weight loss. One study examined a group of participants whose goal was to lose weight and keep it off. These participants were divided into two groups. One group was told to keep a food diary and the other was told to keep track of activity in an exercise diary. According to the results, both groups lost the same amount of weight over time, even though one group kept track of diet and one kept track of exercise.

Another study found that people who are trying to lose weight benefit from distractions, but only if they are enjoyable distractions that don't make them feel guilty or stressed out about their diets.

While we can't guarantee that losing weight is all about calories in and calories out, it is clear that distractions can help to increase the likelihood of weight loss.

Instead of avoiding diet distractions altogether, try using them to your advantage. Diet distractions are things that give you pleasure, but they also can help you lose weight and keep it off. The diet distraction technique works like this: Instead of focusing on what you can't eat, focus on why you can eat certain foods. By asserting this healthy principle, you begin to view yourself as a person who is able to have fun eating and still lose weight. It's like being told that your diet won't allow you to have chocolate chip cookies for lunch but instead allows peanut butter and jelly sandwiches.

When you are thinking about eating "unhealthy" foods, try to dig through your memories and think of other things besides food. Moreover, you can fantasize about your body's inspiration and this can help you get motivated to continue with your diet.

Some people have a rare type of syndrome, they are never short of advice in the form of diet plans and routines that they stick to religiously. But for those who perceive it as challenging to stop themselves from making a food choice when they know deep down inside it's not good for them, this is for you. It will teach you how distraction can help rid your mind of the dangerous thoughts that have been troubling you throughout the day. You will discover that you can conveniently stay disciplined by turning your energy into a plan that is not only healthy but easy to follow. It will help you to remember that your time at the gym and running after food are a small part of life. Accept this fact and let your life be fun and not overweight.

Decide to Improve Your Health

Evidence-based studies suggest that fifteen to twenty percent of Americans suffer from some type of obsessive-compulsive disorder. If you fit into this group, you may find it difficult to be disciplined about your diet when your mind is consumed with thoughts of food and weight loss. If you have already tried many diets, but still haven't found one that works for you, try the distraction technique. Make a list of foods that you can't resist. You need to understand why you are eating the food when you know it's not good for your health. The main reasons include:

- **Feelings of boredom:** Are you consuming foods as a way to avoid work? If this is the circumstance, try to explore other activities that are more interesting and will help keep your mind busy.
- **Emotions:** Do you eat when you are angry or frustrated? If so, use visualization or meditation techniques to deal with these emotions in a positive manner. Remember, distractions are a positive thing, you need to learn to turn them into an advantage so you can discover what you desire in life.
- **Habits:** Do you have bad habits that are destroying your health? If so, it will become easier for you to be disciplined and avoid consuming bad foods. Just instill in your mind that no matter how difficult it is, the power of distraction is there to help you along.

Plan Ahead

If your aim is to stay on top of your weight-loss goals, try not to eat until later in the evening. This will help you to avoid cravings for a late-night snack. This will also help you to eliminate the temptation of snacking in the evening. When you are midday hungry and need something to eat, try eating a small meal that is healthy for your body and doesn't contain too much fat. Your body will be able to accept this small meal and not feel as if you are missing out on anything. While you are eating this light meal, try to read or watch a movie. This will keep your mind occupied with something that is not related to food. If you need more help with keeping your mind off food, try something distracting like listening to loud music or going for a walk. You will find that eating can soon become an easy task when you have the power of distraction working for you! Believe it or not, distraction is a powerful tool in stopping unhealthy habits like this one before they develop. To do it effectively though, there are some things you need to remember about how your brain works and how you should go about implementing these strategies:

Your Mind Can't Multitask Well

The rest of your body is capable of doing many things at once. You can walk, talk, and use your phone or do anything else that requires two or more actions. But your brain is very different. In order to concentrate on multiple things at once, it would have to focus mainly on one task while relying on you or some other source to take care of the others. That means that if you're trying to do several things at once, you're either going to have to be distracted away from the actual task or you're going to end up doing only one thing and missing half of what needs to be done.

Distraction Is a Learned Behavior

Even if it sounds counter-intuitive, being in a state of distraction can actually put you at risk for eating too much. People who tend to experience this often find that when they're doing something else, they can get lost in their thoughts and forget to eat at all. But if you're able to learn how to distract yourself effectively from the urge to eat too much, it will be much easier for you to stop that urge before it takes control of you.

Those who have ever been on a diet know how easy it is to be distracted by delicious food. Your willpower might not hold up against a store full of doughnuts, chocolate bars, and ice cream. We can't blame you; the things we crave are delicious!

The first action that you can perform is to find healthy distractions like reading a book or doing some DIY projects or puzzles.

One of the most important distractions you can use for avoiding overeating is exercise. Even though it may seem like you are just doing something extra, it is in fact helpful in more ways than one. Workouts like yoga or walking will not only help you to burn a ton of calories, but it will also aid in relieving stress and take your mind off food. It's important when doing an intense workout to stick with the routine so your body has the time and energy to get rid of toxins that are present throughout your day.

One way to avoid overeating is to make a conscious effort about the food you eat. When you start thinking about why you're eating, it can really limit your consumption. This allows you to eat in moderation while still getting the nutrients that your body needs. One thing to do is to write in a food journal.

At the end of each day, write down everything that you ate for breakfast, lunch, dinner, and snacks. Take note of every detail and how much you ate. By doing this, you can see the simple changes that you can make in the way you eat. It may seem like a lot of work, but it's well worth it!

Finally, one of the best ways to get rid of those cravings is to drink water when they come around. When your body is dehydrated, your cravings will get worse. You can avoid this by drinking water before going to bed at night and having it during the day as well. This will help you maintain a healthy body weight and keep your cravings under control.

An effective way to avoid overeating is something that will help you stay relaxed. Stress and anxiety often lead to cravings, so the best way to avoid overeating or reaching for food is by keeping a positive attitude all the time.

CHAPTER 4:

Do Not Postpone the Pleasure

Many people try to get in shape by postponing their favorite foods in favor of bland and slightly more healthy options. If you're like me, you probably haven't read about the science behind how hormones impact mood or energy levels, which are two factors that are commonly cited when people decide that they want to lose weight. Let's take a look at some research on this topic.

The Nature of Desire

It's common knowledge that desire and expectations are two factors that can influence people's experience in a given situation. In a 2010 investigation, researchers wanted to find out whether or not an image of a desired object would make that object more appealing.

The researchers had people look at images of a bracelet and then rate how much they wanted the bracelet. As you can see, there was a clear difference between those who saw the image of the bracelet and those who hadn't. All participants in the study experienced a decrease in desire after seeing the image of the desired object, but only those participants who were primed to want to have that item rated the object as less appealing than those participants who were not primed to want it. Participants from both groups rated their desire for having something at its initial level, but all showed greater increases in their desire upon exposure to an image of that item.

This study suggests that simply wanting something will increase your desire for that thing. It is essential to remember, however, that individuals who are primed to want an object (whether or not they actually want it) rate the object as less appealing than subjects who are not primed to want it. That is, while the first group did report less desire when looking at an image of the desired item, they still rated it as more attractive than those who were not primed to want it. It seems that even when an object is appealing, having a desire for it can decrease how appealing you think that object is.

The Pleasure of Pursuit

Another study, from 2006, looked at the impact of desire regarding achievement. In this case, research subjects were asked to listen to either a sad piece of music or a happy song before playing Tetris on a computer. The researchers found that those participants who listened to happier music rated their experience as more satisfying after finishing the game than those who listened to sad music before playing. However, the researchers also found that people who listened to happy music showed more desire for playing the game than those who listened to sad music. In this case, it seems that desiring something increased a person's pleasure from achieving that goal.

What About Weight Loss?

While the former two studies show us how desire can influence our experience of a given activity, they do not help us to understand how our desires can impact our long-term health and wellness. Therefore, let's take a look at a study on dieting which helps us to see how our desire to achieve a goal can impact whether or not that goal is achieved.

In this experiment, published in the Journal of Consumer Research in 2009 by Alan J. Sanfey and James K. Rilling, participants were asked about their desire for food during different moments of their day. In each case, the researchers found that participants' desires for food were highest immediately before meals and lowest immediately after meals. In addition, people who experience decreased desires for food were more likely to consume that food than those who did not. Sanfey and Rilling attribute this effect to the fact that people with decreased desires for food have less control over choosing what they eat and when they eat it. Their current conditions of hunger or satiety influence their ability to control the foods they choose to eat in these instances.

The Desire for Something

While all of the data suggest that desires can and do influence how we feel about things in our lives, it's important to remember that desires are never static. Research from 2012 shows that many of us experience a desire for something (which may or may not be food) just before reaching the final stages of weight loss (which often coincide with the appearance of weight loss). In this study, which was published in Psychological Science by David M. Rosenbaum and Roxanne M. Cason, researchers found that weight-loss participants who had lost less than twenty percent of their desired weight showed no difference in desire for food before and after a meal. However, those who had lost twenty percent or more of their original body weight had significantly less desire for food before the meal than those who had lost less than twenty percent of their body weight. The researchers suggest that as a result of reaching their goal weight, these participants' bodies were already beginning to experience satiety before the meal!

So, while our desire for things (even food) may be strong, that desire can change over time or as we achieve our goals. Hence, it is crucial to remember that part of your goal does not have to include eating less than you want. Instead, you may want to think about what your long-term goals are and how your desire for something will affect those goals.

It's widely known that being overweight can be unhealthy, in addition to making you feel less confident and/or more self-conscious. But did you know that by eating less often, or postponing pleasure to lose weight, you could actually gain weight?

There are plenty of warnings about skipping meals and overdoing it on low-calorie food. The idea of eating less to lose weight is nothing new but the effect this approach has on how you feel.

Eating less often is an effective way for people to lose weight because they will burn more calories overall by doing so. Someone who lives in the United States, for example, would need to consume about 2,100 calories a day if they want to maintain their current weight. But if they eat less often, they can burn up to 300 additional calories a day (just from the extra work their body has to do to digest food).

The main problem with eating less often is that it doesn't give your body time to adapt. When you first start skipping meals, you'll probably feel hungry and lightheaded because your body hasn't yet adjusted to the change. That's why it's not a good idea to take this approach immediately and without preparation.

Instead, you should gradually start eating less often by eliminating one or two meals each week. This will allow your body to adjust slowly to the new changes. And once your body is used to it, it'll be easier for you to stick with what you're doing because your body won't fight against the changes as much.

But other problems can occur when someone starts eating less often. The main one is that it can make your body try to store more calories than usual. This means it will take longer for you to lose weight. And since your body doesn't know how to deal with these sudden changes, it could end up being a lot harder for you to "adapt."

To avoid this problem, you should try not to eat less more than three times a week. And when you do, make sure you don't skip meals. Instead, try to spread out your low-calorie days throughout the week and always try to have a meal at midday.

Another thing you should avoid is skipping meals to lose weight. The idea that you'll get hungrier over time (or feel uncomfortable because your body doesn't know when it's supposed to eat again) might sound like a good way of motivating you to eat less. But it isn't.

According to recent research, this approach can actually backfire on you and make you give up on your goals. Why? Because your body will learn to adjust to the changes by sending out strong hunger signals whenever it's about to be hungry (or when it's time for you to eat again). This is why it can be an effective way of losing weight.

But when you go to eat less often, your body will send out strong hunger signals—even though it's not actually hungry. And if you ignore these signals and lose weight by eating less, your body could end up getting stuck in a pattern of "feeling hungry all the time." It will end up thinking eating more often is what it needs to do to maintain your current weight.

So instead of approaching over-eating by skipping meals, you should try to approach it by consuming more calories overall each day. If you do this, it won't be as difficult for you to lose weight.

CHAPTER 5:

Discover the True Meaning of Hunger

A person is hungry when in the absence of sufficient food to meet the body's needs, chemical reactions resulting in a low blood sugar level cause hunger. Hunger is a significant and often unpleasant sensory state experienced as a feeling of emptiness or lack. Hormones such as leptin and ghrelin also play roles in regulating appetite. The experience of hunger is closely related to the body's nutritional status.

Hunger can be an overwhelming sensation resulting in loss of decision-making and self-control, known as "psychophagy," or in an increased desire to eat, known as hyperphagia. In extreme cases, hunger can cause people to inflict harm on others for food. Compulsive eating disorders are a form of psychological addiction; psychological addiction is characterized by compulsive engagement in rewarding stimuli that have negative consequences.

According to proponents of the dopamine hypothesis of reward, hunger is a motivational state that evolved from the need to satisfy needs for food to survive. In this view, there is pleasure associated with eating but no instinctive drive for food. People who eat when they are not hungry or overeat are said to be over-consumers.

In other hypotheses, the experience of hunger may have evolved from a need for nutrients and energy in order to grow and develop. In this view, the subjective experience of hunger is a biological imperative triggered by the need to gain energy from food. This need for nutrients and energy can be satisfied with food even in the absence of any conscious desire to eat.

Historically, hunger has been a major cause of starvation, which kills approximately 1 billion people per year. With rapid advances in agricultural technology and increasing urbanization, hunger is becoming rarer in modern times. Scientifically controlled methods of producing food also have led to a dramatic rise in the food supply.

In developed countries, food waste is often thrown out with the trash, even though it could have been consumed by humans or animals. According to a study by Natural Resources Defense Council and Harvard University Law School's Food Law and Policy Clinic, 40% of Americans' food goes uneaten every year. The same study claims that "between 30–40% of all fruit, vegetable and grain produce grown annually in the U.S. is not consumed at all, and a much greater percentage is lost or wasted along the distribution chain from farm to fork."

Hunger is an innate need that has been present since the dawn of humanity. The first recorded recordings of humans feeling hungry were found in the writings of Aristotle. These early records suggested that hunger was a natural part of life and did not indicate any sense of suffering or guilt associated with hunger.

Hunger is a desire for food and drinks that can drive a person to eat or drink even when not hungry. Most commonly, these are called digestive functions but they also occur for the brain in a state of rest. Hunger is an instinctive feeling with no rational basis, and during times of famine, it may be difficult or impossible to ignore this need as it can result in death by starvation if left unfulfilled.

Hunger From Anger

Hunger from anger is a condition where one's hunger increases while experiencing anger due to the dopamine release that comes with the fight or flight response. This can be caused by various factors including periods of no food intake, dieting, and stress. If you aren't getting enough sleep and you become angry, your brain may think that since you have been fighting for too long for energy purposes, more food is needed. The result is hunger from an anger episode.

The underlying cause of extreme anger in the human body can be traced to the hypothalamus, which is the controlling center located inside of our brain stem. The hypothalamus is responsible for regulating basic functions such as eating behavior and sleeping patterns. When you are hungry or you've been awake for a long period of time, your body will send signals to your hypothalamus to activate your "fight or flight" response and help regulate these basic biological functions. In addition to these basic biological functions, the hypothalamus also regulates your emotions like anger. When activated, this area of your brain will send out signals to your sympathetic nervous system which then triggers the release of endorphins; hormones that enhance your mood and make you feel good.

For the reasons mentioned above, it is no surprise that when we're angry we experience a feeling of increased hunger.

The solution to this type of emotion is not to suppress or try too hard to control it, but rather be aware of its presence and know-how to deal with the situation. Namely, you must be able to stop yourself from reacting violently towards people in a negative way. If you were going through a period of extreme anger, you should let go of the anger or don't even react in the first place.

This can be achieved by doing certain things in your daily life to keep yourself from getting angry.

One way you can do this is to follow a strict diet so that you are not hungry. Another option is to get enough sleep and exercise regularly so that you can control your emotions better.

Hunger From Apathy

Apathy is the state of not caring enough to get things done. It's a lack of interest in life and more specifically in the things you do. Hunger is a feeling that leads to apathy, while hunger from apathy is given by an individual that has not been taking care of themselves. For some people, apathy can also be associated with melancholy or depression.

Apathy can be caused by numerous reasons. The most obvious cause is sadness and depression. Sadness and depression often cause someone to lose interest in their life or the things they once loved doing. It's hard to want to do something when you are sad, depressed, or even angry because sadness and happiness are two polar opposites of each other.

This reason can be more complicated than it looks at first glance. The causes of apathy can be determined by looking at two main factors: the relationship someone has with their environment, and with themselves.

The first factor for apathy is how you view your surroundings. What you think of the people around you and where you live in general will influence your actions. This is because if you are unhappy or frustrated with where you live, it will be hard to like living there. A good environment will make you happier and boost your confidence. A bad one will make you angry and negative.

The second factor for apathy is how people view themselves. Someone can get apathetic when they believe that they are not pretty or interesting enough. This is mainly because they feel as though no one will like them if they are not popular or talked about. This is called social pressure. People tend to get apathetic when they are insecure about themselves.

Hunger from apathy is a type of hunger that is caused by delaying the effects of hunger so that it is not noticeable enough for the person to become aware of it. It's when a person acts out in ways they normally would not, because they want to put off symptoms and make them worth waiting for. Hunger from apathy is different from hunger for other forms of hunger. The person does not want to grow close to the people they care about and will ignore them if they don't seem interested in the things the individual wants to do. Hunger from apathy can make someone feel as though there isn't enough time in the world for them and that no matter how hard they work, it won't be enough. They will slowly lose themselves until they become apathetic.

Hunger for Suffering

The feeling of hunger is an unpleasant sensation that is unfulfilled and requires more to satiate it. Hunger can also be described as the longing for spiritual or psychological pain. It is a spiritual desire for something which has not yet been experienced, and thus experiencing it would make one feel fulfilled. The opposite of hunger, nurturance, would create the absence of this sensation. Nurturing creates relief from hunger in its higher-level meanings because nourishing encourages possibilities of growth and change while preventing stagnation within oneself.

CHAPTER 6:

Bring Out the Real Yourself

You know that feeling when you look in the mirror and are disappointed with what you see? You know, when the fat is spilling out of your clothes and your skin looks sallow and pasty? That's not how it has to be. Put weight loss into action and know how to lose weight. You can do it!

Don't allow the extra weight to control you. It's a struggle to be overweight so don't give up and let it take over your life. If you are not contented with how much you weigh, you have the power to change that. You can transform it easily, so try using these methods for losing weight:

- **Weight-loss workout:** Aerobics exercise will help tone up muscles and lose weight. It is an effective way to lose weight. A great workout is 3 sets of 10–12 repetitions of each exercise with a few minutes break. If you want to lose some pounds off, you have to be stronger and leaner than your current body size.
- **Weight-loss diet:** You can try this! The point is to do exercises daily or as much as possible for at least half an hour a day.
- **Meals to consume and foods to avoid in your weight-loss diet.** Drink at least 1.5 liters of water per day. Avoid junk food, soft drinks, burgers, pizza, cakes, etc. Instead, eat lots of fruits and vegetables (corn is good).

- **Avoid stress as much as possible.** Execute relaxation techniques such as yoga, meditation, or breathing exercises every day for 15–20 minutes. Remove all the clutter from your room or house. It will help you to concentrate on what you are doing.
- **Sleep better.** Get your sleep at least 7 hours a day.
- **Declutter your mind.** Go for a walk and use the time to think about things positively.
- **Exercise:** Always remember that exercise is as important as dieting to lose weight fast. You can execute most of the exercises at your residence as long as you have weights or dumbbells at hand. Try to take small steps and if possible, find a buddy who will help you with motivation and correct the position of muscles while exercising.

As we all know, being overweight can affect anyone's life drastically in a negative manner, and this can be seen in many different fields of expertise. If you are one of those people who are constantly struggling to lose weight, then it is time for you to read this article! So, let's start right away.

Many of us do not have the willpower to ignore cravings for foods that are high in calories. If you find yourself eating one meal a day, then you should try increasing the portion size of all your meals so you will be less hungry and thus less likely to fall prey to eating everything that is within your reach. This will aid you to acquire power over your food cravings so that you can stop overeating.

People who don't know how to include exercise into their daily existence may have a hard time sticking to a healthy diet plan. If you are one of those people trying your best to watch what you eat, but find yourself skipping out on exercise, then it is time for you to start learning the value of exercise. You will be happier and healthier if you include exercise in your life.

If you feel that you are too tired to exercise, then it is time for you to try some aerobic exercises. Aerobic exercises can make your heart rate increase and this will make you sweat a lot. This will also help improve your sense of well-being, and all of these benefits can be enjoyed in little time spent.

Your Self-Image Is Your Self-Fulfilling Prophecy

"She didn't know it couldn't be done, so she went ahead and did it."—Mary Almanac.

The concept of your self-image: the way you perceive and define yourself. You will constantly live up to your self-image; it's what you truly believe about yourself. If you have a low self-image regarding your weight and you are attempting to lose weight, it's almost guaranteed that it's not going to happen. Even if you do somehow lose the weight for a while, you'll self-sabotage and put all the weight back on in order to match the image you hold of yourself. You can try "dieting" all you want, but you'll never experience a lasting change until you first change your self-image.

Of course, the opposite is also true. Once you evolve and your self-image becomes that of a fit person at your ideal weight, you'll naturally begin to lose pounds and inches. This is because you will begin to automatically think about how your positive self-image thinks, and, as a result, you'll make the right healthy choices over and over again.

How do you see yourself? What do you believe about yourself? What type of person are you? What are you capable of? I'm not asking who you say you are, or who you would like to be.

Let's go much deeper. I'm asking you, who do you honestly believe you are right now?

And I'm asking this because you are much more than you currently realize or believe you are. We both know this. And I'm also asking because, interestingly enough, research confirms over and over again that who you think you are, affects you more than anything else. Your self-image is a self-fulfilling prophecy. It defines every single limit and boundary and identity cornerstone in your life. It matters more than your level of education, your parent's influence, the town you grew up in, and the schools you went to. It is your thinking that conceives your reality; it's all based on your beliefs about yourself and the world around you. Who you think you are—and what you think you are capable of—defines every limit and boundary and identity cornerstone in your life?

So, who are you? Are you a person who tackles and completes whatever you decide to do? Or do you believe you are a person who doesn't follow through? In life, you're going to end up getting the results that you believe you're going to get. This is especially true in regard to weight loss. If you believe, on some level, that you're a person who will be always struggling with your weight ... then you will be. If you believe that you lack willpower or the determination to evolve into the next best version of yourself, how do you think your actions and results will compare with those of people who know they are ready to change their eating habits, their weight, and their lives?

Pause and take a look at yourself. You bought this book with a specific outcome in mind. Now examine your level of involvement in this book and program up until now. Have you been taking this book seriously? Have you been fully participating in the exercises? Have you been online watching the accompanying videos? Have you chosen a weight-loss buddy? Have you been on a "detox"? I ask because all of these things are determined by your beliefs and self-image.

Never forget that you're the master of your fate. Believing in yourself means discovering, evaluating, and rewriting your old, limiting beliefs. Alter your thoughts and you alter your world. This is because we act upon our beliefs as if they are true and make our decisions based on these beliefs. We continually seek out validation and evidence of our beliefs through our experiences, further validating them. It's a self-feeding cycle that makes our beliefs our reality...

Belief is the "secret sauce" of all transformation. So, what do you believe—and how much thought have you given it? This is something I highly encourage you to invest your time and energy in; it's imperative if you want to achieve sustainable weight loss. Separate your beliefs into two categories:

1. **How things are.** This is your construct of the world and how it operates. It's the lens or filters you see and experience everything through.
2. **How you are.** These are your beliefs about yourself; what you think you're capable of doing or being.

CHAPTER 7:

The 3 Things That Keep You From Getting Back in Shape

Perfectionism

"I am a perfectionist when it comes to my diet."

This statement is representative of how many people try to control their lives, but it can lead to self-sabotage. It is important to examine what drives your behavior so that you can adjust accordingly. In doing so, you will find lasting success without any more of the stress or regretful outcomes associated with unhealthy eating habits.

The Role of Perfectionism in Dieting

For some, perfectionism is an integral part of their personality. They are never satisfied with themselves or their accomplishments. They compare their selves to other individuals and feel like they come up short; perfectionism is their constant companion. Having a sense of perfectionism can be an advantageous characteristic in some circumstances, such as when striving for academic excellence. However, for many people, perfectionism is not helpful or necessary. Those with this personality trait believe that a perfect outcome is essential for them to be satisfied. They focus on what's rather than who's in a situation, and when they are not reaching their goal, it becomes very difficult for them to stop thinking about it. One of the reasons why perfectionism influences dieting is because dieting often involves striving for goals like losing weight, building muscle, or gaining more energy. These goals can be tough to achieve, especially because it is often difficult to stick with specific diets and exercise programs. Dieting can bring about feelings of self-doubt and lack of confidence. Perfectionism can bring up feelings of frustration, disappointment in oneself or others, and insecurity. If an individual has perfectionist tendencies, he or she may begin to feel like a failure when they are unable or unwilling to reach their goal. This will lead to a state of depression and negative emotions such as anger, sadness, anxiety, or withdrawal.

What Is Perfectionism?

Perfectionism has been defined as a desire to appear and be perfect, with the need for everyone else to meet the same high standards. Most people who strive for perfection do so to achieve success and achieve their goals. They think that they are more likely to succeed when they work harder and are more careful. While perfectionism is a normal part of most people's lives, extreme levels of perfectionism can make it difficult to function normally. People who struggle with extreme levels of perfectionism are more likely to struggle with depression and other forms of emotional distress.

Why Does Perfectionism Play a Role in Dieting?

When people are trying to change their eating habits, they often find that their old habits come back into play. For example, if a person is trying to lose weight, she may be tempted to eat junk food or binge on foods he or she knows are not good for him or her. This can be a downer for someone who is trying hard to change his or her behavior. Below is a list of some well-known reasons why people with perfectionist tendencies might be at risk for bingeing and restricting when dieting.

- **Perfectionism makes it difficult to be open about their eating habits:** People with perfectionist tendencies often have difficulty discussing their negative feelings or behavior. Because they see themselves as the perfect person, they don't want to risk being found out as being imperfect or having bad habits. They may feel like their secret will be revealed.

- **Perfectionism makes it difficult to ask for help:** Asking for help is not very easy for perfectionists. They want to be sure that they can handle the situation on their own and do not want to risk having their weaknesses exposed.

- **Perfectionism makes change difficult:** People who are perfectionists fear failure. They would rather avoid making changes in the first place than risk failure when they do so.

- **Perfectionists are often afraid to enjoy life:** While perfectionists feel that they must always strive for perfection, they also feel guilty when they allow themselves to enjoy life. They believe that enjoying life will lower their standards.

- **Perfectionists often have a need for control:** People who struggle with perfectionism have a need to be in control of every situation. They fear making changes because it upsets the order that they have created in their lives and makes them more vulnerable to criticism or failure.

How Does Perfectionism Affect Dieting?

When perfectionists attempt to change their eating habits, they often find it difficult or impossible to be successful. It is important to understand that perfectionism can make it difficult to stick with a healthy diet. If you have a propensity toward perfectionism, you may find your efforts are frustrated by sabotaging thoughts and feelings.

To make lasting changes with your diet, you must be able to develop healthy strategies for coping with perfectionism. Here are a few actions that you can do to change the way you deal with perfectionist thinking.

- **Accept your feelings:** Perfectionism is a common personality trait that is part of who you are. You may have difficulty accepting this fact because it makes you feel "less than" perfect. Remember that everyone has flaws and when you accept your flaws it will help you accept others.

- **Make a point to be aware of your feelings:** You can't control what you feel. But you can learn to recognize how your feelings affect your thinking and behavior. When you identify the thoughts that trigger perfectionist thinking, you have the opportunity to develop better-coping skills.

- **Stop putting yourself down:** Don't judge yourself for not being perfect. Rather, think about how great you have come when it comes to changing your behavior or diet.

False Goals

It's not uncommon for people who are trying to lose weight to have some sort of goal in mind, but it's important to make sure that those goals are realistic.

Keeping a realistic goal means that you can achieve a reasonable outcome without too much work or stress. Unrealistic goals, on the other hand, might set you up for failure from the start. What's worse is when unrealistic expectations become your reality because then they start dictating how you perceive all your future dieting efforts.

If your desire is to lose some pounds, start by setting realistic goals. It's also a great approach to make sure that you have some small amount of weight-loss success under your belt. This will give you a benchmark to measure your progress against so that when you reach the big goal, the results will seem even more satisfying.

Here are some simple guidelines for setting realistic goals:

- **Make sure that you choose a weight-loss goal that is bigger than you think you can achieve.** This will give you the motivation to work at it. If your goal seems too easy, then it's not challenging and you may become bored and quit. You can always adjust your goal once you've had some success with it.
- **Be realistic about how much weight you'll lose within a specific period of time.** For example, if you want to shed off 10 pounds in under one month, don't set your goal at a weight loss of 10 pounds per week. You might only be able to lose those 5 pounds after a month and then the motivation might lessen.

- **Be certain that you have realistic expectations about how much weight you need to lose.** Sometimes people are discouraged by the amount of weight they see written on the scale, but if you calculate your daily weight loss, then you can adjust for items such as activity level or water intake.
- **If you gain some weight back after reaching your goal, then it's not the end of the world.** Even though it's frustrating and disappointing, you can continue to work toward achieving your goal.
- **Don't set yourself up for failure by making unrealistic goals.** The only way you will achieve them is if you are determined to succeed. Set a timeline for your goals and make sure that you are realistic about how long it will take before you achieve them.

The Judgement of Others

It's unlikely that you've ever met anyone who likes being judged. We all have insecurities, and there's nothing like someone pointing them out for us to feel like our world is crumbling. That's why it's so heartbreaking when good friends turn on their own friends through negative comments made in the presence of others about things, they do to take care of themselves.

For example, you may have a friend who has decided to go on a diet but no one finds it necessary to remind her that she needs to lose weight. Instead, people say things like what she's wearing is "too tight" or that you can tell she gained weight. You may even be guilty of doing this yourself.

When we start judging the way our close friends take care of themselves it discourages them from seeking support for their journeys and often makes them feel bad about themselves.

The sad thing is that it's easy to make comments without even realizing it. It usually happens when our emotional selves are in overdrive and we're not aware of what we're saying or how it might come across.

When this happens, it's more constructive to ask for clarification before dropping the bomb on someone you care about. You may even find that the person you're speaking to is not choosing the way they are taking care of themselves.

For example, you may be angry at your friend because she's never able to hang out with you due to work and family obligations. It just happens that she's decided to switch from fast food to home-cooked meals as a way to make her life healthier.

You might not know this, and, because you're frustrated with her being unavailable, you may see her healthy choices as a way to make yourself feel better about the fact that she can't make time for you. Instead of judging her, just be sympathetic and offer to help where you can.

If you're on the receiving end of judgment while trying to lose weight, avoid justifying your choices. Instead, think about how you want to be treated. Are you trying to become a better person for everyone around you? Of course, it's necessary to take care of yourself without pushing your body so far that you become unhealthy and risk death.

You just might find that the people who criticize you the most are actually jealous because they're struggling with their issues involving weight and don't have the courage to do something about it.

The more you educate yourself on issues surrounding health, the more helpful you'll be to your friends. Instead of allowing others to make judgments for you, learn to accept criticism with a grain of salt and make choices that are best for you.

Don't let a lack of education or knowledge affect your ability to make healthy decisions. Instead, educate yourself and let your choices be an inspiration to others who are struggling with issues surrounding weight loss.

CHAPTER 8:

Address the Right Phrases

Thoughts may seem harmless enough. Outside of characters in comic book movies, we can't move objects with our thoughts, conjure up money with our minds, or read what another person is thinking. At a basic chemical level, a thought is just a tiny spark of electrical activity produced by neurons firing in our brain. The truth is that our thinking patterns do have great power over the quality of our lives. Only, instead of producing an immediate or direct effect on the world around us, thoughts work indirectly by translating from electrical activity in our brain to decisions, actions, and habits that shape our lives and bodies. Briefly stated, our self-talk initiates a domino effect that eventually becomes our lifestyle, and this process molds the state of our body and the quality of our lives over time. The supermarket entrepreneur, Frank Outlaw, eloquently expressed this mental domino effect as follows:

Watch your thoughts, for they become your words.
Watch your words, for they become your actions.
Watch your actions, for they become your habits.
Watch your habits, for they become your character.
Watch your character, for it becomes your destiny.

Thoughts do not have immediate effects on the appearance or weight of our bodies. They shape our bodies slowly by nudging our countless little decisions about food, exercise, sleep, stress, and other health-related factors in a cumulatively favorable or unfavorable direction. Here is why that matters so much: For months, you make literally thousands of seemingly inconsequential decisions that affect your health. Although a single or small number of these health decisions will probably not have a large effect on your weight, multiply this effect by the power of thousands of health decisions over time and you will obtain dramatically different results. A drop of water will not harm you, but if thousands of water drops accumulated over you, you could drown. One of the most important discoveries in the field of psychology over the past century is that differences in how people think explain why some people succeed even at endeavors with high rates of failure. For example, in Napoleon Hill's, Think and Grow Rich, he describes how financially successful people think differently than people that struggle with money. In Martin Seligman's, Learned Optimism, he describes how optimistic people think differently than people that are more pessimistic (leading to very different quality of life outcomes). In John Maxwell's books on leadership, (such as The 21 Irrefutable Laws of Leadership), he describes some of the distinctive thinking patterns common to successful leaders. In sports psychology books, such as Jim Afremow's, *The Champion's Mind*, certain patterns of thinking are shown to contribute to elite athletic performance, and in Carol Dweck's, *Mindset*, she describes how people that persevere and grow from adversity (those with a growth mindset) think differently than people who give up quickly and internalize failures (those with a fixed mindset). Across area after area, certain patterns of thinking separate those that flourish from those that fail. A theme common to all the above areas is that the thinking patterns linked to greater achievement can be learned by a person determined to succeed. I hope that it does not surprise you at this point to learn that thinking patterns contribute just as strongly to success with weight loss.

Let's now look at some specific ways how good and not so good weight managers think that influences the results they obtain.

Before I show you some of these self-talk examples directly, however, I first would like to assess your ideas on the subject with several questions.

I ask you to give each of the four questions below a minute or two of thought before we move on to potentially help you recognize some of the self-talk that you may already engage in that is helping or hindering your weight-loss efforts:

1. How do you imagine people that manage their weight well over time think?
2. How do their patterns of thinking differ from people that struggle with their weight?
3. How can a person that struggles with their weight learn how to think like a thinner and fitter person?
4. How do people with good weight management skills think?

When you appreciate that the quality of our lives closely reflects what we think about most of the time, it makes sense that people who are able to consistently maintain a healthy weight and lifestyle think differently than others.

The figure below provides several examples of how successful weight managers think that translates into the results they enjoy.

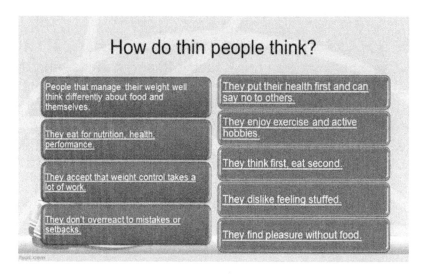

Successful long-term weight managers have a fundamentally different mental orientation to food than others, namely a health orientation rather than a pleasure orientation. Although good weight managers appreciate the taste of food as much as any other person, their primary value system for the kind of diet they follow consistently is how it contributes to their health and their health-related quality of life goals. They similarly think about the process of weight loss and weight management differently; specifically, they have adopted a version of the journey mentality where a long-term commitment of time and effort are considered investments in the weight-loss success they desire. Successful weight managers think of setbacks such as weight regain or dietary lapses as temporary setbacks, solvable problems, tests of their resolve, or as learning opportunities. They recognize that the process of losing weight and improving their fitness requires some hardships and sacrifices along the way and see these experiences as the price to pay for the cherished reward of reaching their goals. Finally, successful weight managers don't think of eating as a way to manage stress, reward themselves, or as being their central source of enjoyment at social events and holidays. Imagine a hypothetical person with the pattern of food and exercise-related thinking described in this figure. If you knew nothing else about them, what would you guess about their weight and health status?

How Do People That Struggle With Their Weight Think?

Now let's look at the alternative: examples of the food and exercise thinking patterns that poorer weight managers tend to experience. Looking at the figure below, you can see that differences in thinking between this group and the former thinner and fitter group are dramatic. Rather than as fuel for their health goals, people that struggle with their weight typically prioritize the taste and pleasure components of the foods they eat, including often eating for emotional reasons. They eat in a way consistent with the usually unhealthy ways that they think about themselves (the healthy identity effect in reverse). They react to hunger pains as if they are emergencies, leading them to make food choices based on convenience and leaving them vulnerable to cravings induced by advertising and environmental cues. For many people that struggle with their weight, the act of eating their favorite foods is like spending time in a comfortable relationship that reduces emotional pain and produces emotional pleasure. For many otherwise lonely people, food has become their best friend. Finally, people in the overweight group are more impulsive in their thinking and decision making about food: the immediate gratification from food is more valued than the long-term effects, and the consequences of their food choices are considered only after the food is consumed (often when the guilt kicks in). Once again, if you knew nothing more about a person than that their thinking patterns about food and exercise resembled those in the figure below, you would have little difficulty guessing that they struggle to maintain a healthy weight.

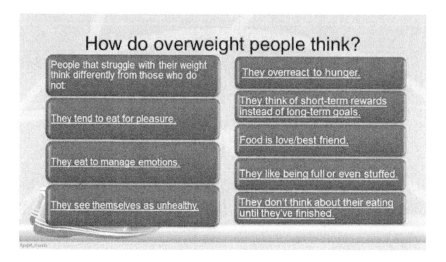

How old were you and where were you when you decided to think and talk to yourself as you do now? Although you likely learned many lessons from your parents and your teachers in school, were you ever taught how to think effectively? For most people, the answers to these questions are never and no. Instead, the way that most of us learned to think was like the haphazard method a bird uses to make a nest: by picking up whatever happened to be in the area at the time.

Why do you (probably) speak English as your native language instead of another language? This was probably not because you sampled the many languages available and consciously chose English as the language that was most useful for you. Even though you were born with the biological capacity to learn any language spoken in the world, you learned to speak

English because, mostly by chance, English was the language spoken by the people around you. Had you been born at another time, in another country, or with parents that spoke a different language, then you might now not even be able to understand English. The point here is that much of how you communicate with others and with yourself was determined by luck and by factors mostly out of your control. If your luck happened to be bad in this regard, then it has put you in a difficult position to be successful in your life.

But here is another way of considering this: even though it may have been due mostly to the chance that you speak English if you wanted to learn a new language now, such as Spanish or French, at your current age and in your current circumstances, could you? And if you could learn a new language to help you communicate more effectively to others, isn't it also possible that you could learn to communicate more effectively to yourself? The answer to both questions is yes, and that puts us back in the driver's seat of our communication habits if we are willing to take the wheel. Even if you picked up some ineffective thinking patterns from your parents or role models when growing up, it is never too late to turn the process around.

Although your relationships with other people can make a big difference to your weight-loss goals, there is just one relationship upon which your goal of long-term weight loss depends entirely: your relationship with yourself. Your journey to a healthy weight can be assisted in many ways by supportive friends and family or by working with skilled health professionals. However, none of these relationships will be enough to achieve your long-term goal of a healthy weight until you learn to become a friend to yourself. A self-relationship based on self-criticism, negative emotions, and seeing the worst in yourself will doom even the best weight-loss program to eventual failure and prevent you from enjoying any results that you manage to obtain along the way.

CHAPTER 9:

Enough With Self-Abuse

What Not to Say

The struggle with our weight is often an ongoing battle. Sometimes, it can feel like we have tried everything to lose weight and yet still find ourselves gaining a few pounds each day. We eat well and exercise, but our progress is stagnant at best—and hopeless when we fall off the wagon a bit. No matter what you do, it seems to find the right diet that works for you is impossible. As if it isn't hard enough to stick to a diet, many people also have to contend with that nagging voice in their head. That self-sabotaging inner monologue is one of the main reasons why people give up on diets—they can't stand listening to that voice.

It's actually essential for us to listen to our thoughts. They help us understand who we are and differentiate between right and wrong, true and false, healthy and unhealthy. They help us deal with our emotions, and with many aspects of life. We are better off when we learn to control our thoughts rather than being controlled by them. But not all thoughts are helpful or useful. We must listen to the voice in our head, but we should be selective in what we listen to and whom we listen to.

The thoughts are the process of self-talk or speaking to yourself. It can be accomplished out loud or silently. There are two types of self-talk: negative and positive. Negative self-talk helps no one. It's unhelpful, unproductive, and just plain depressing. It's why so many people sabotage their diets by talking themselves out of it—they don't think they can do it so they won't even try. The positive kind, however, allows us to stay focused and do what we need to do to get the results we're looking for.

So how do we get our negative thoughts to step aside and let the positive ones take their place? It's actually pretty easy—we only have to wait for new thoughts to come into our minds. Since negative thoughts are all around us, they'll enter your mind more often than you think. You may not even acknowledge it at first, but you are most likely already have some in your head! These thoughts may be mild at first but can grow and become more frequent as time goes on. The more you hear these negative thoughts, the more they'll become a problem.

You can deal with negative thoughts the same way you deal with a bully—ignore them! If a bad person were to come up to you and yell insults in your face, what would you do? You'd most likely tell the person off. But if instead of yelling at you, the bully walked past you while muttering insults under his breath, it wouldn't be as offensive. Likely, the initial action that you need to do when you hear a negative thought is to ignore it! The more you try to think about it, the more your mind will replay it and the more negative thoughts will come up to torment you. You need to get that voice out of your head.

Just like a bully, a negative thought can't hurt us if we don't listen to it. We don't get upset when the bully yells insults at us because we know he's not really worth being angry about. The same is true for negative thoughts. If you're trying to lose weight, the voice in your head will inevitably say things like, "I can't do it," or "This diet is impossible." These are all real thoughts that we all have at some point. When we hear them, however, we need to respond with "I don't believe that. I can do it." Just like telling a bully-off, you'll need to say that to yourself in a confident tone. The words themselves don't matter; the tone of your voice is what matters most.

The only solution you can do to rid of negative thoughts is by replacing them with something else. That's why it's important to consciously choose what to think about. We can't stop the negative thoughts from coming in, but we can decide not to listen to them and instead focus on something more positive. For example, the first thing a new dieter needs to do is change what they're thinking. They need to start with something that's completely positive, something that will be easy to keep on track. You can't lose weight if you don't want to—so you need to start with that.

Nothing wrong with starting with self-talk in general, but it's better if you begin by talking about what you want to happen—not what you don't want to happen. You don't want to lose weight; you want to be healthy and look good. You don't want to eat that extra piece of cake; you want to eat more healthy foods and get better results from your workouts. You can't take away the negative thoughts without adding something positive.

We all have our own opinions in our minds. They're as unique as we are—that's why they seem so different from everyone else's minds. But that's not necessarily bad at all! We all have the capacity for greatness. This is special because it's yours and yours alone. The power to change your life and be positive lies in that voice. You can take control of it like no one else can, you're the only one who can change what you think and how powerful those thoughts are.

We sometimes can't see our own mistakes, but the voice in our heads will constantly guide us. So, if that voice is negative, we need to make it positive. We need to create a new one. It may take time and it may be hard at first, but you can do it! And when you do, you'll finally start making your dreams come true.

Positive Affirmations

At the heart of thought, power is the notion that your thoughts create your collective circumstances and conditions. Every aspect of your present life, be it relationships, finances, health, or self-image, is the offspring of your most common thoughts and the feelings, emotions, and beliefs they create.

You are not your circumstance; you create your circumstances whatever they may be, wanted or unwanted. The simplest way to create thought awareness is to accept the truth that, through their unlimited creative power, your thoughts create your circumstances, and therefore, by being aware of the most common thoughts in your mind, you can determine which thoughts/seeds to cultivate and care for thereby changing your reality or circumstances.

To create thought awareness, look within yourself as your reality begins in your mind. Only by being alive to your mind can you create thought awareness. Only by being aware of the energy created by specific and common thoughts can you change the attendant energy in specific areas of your life.

Your dominant habits, your beliefs, and mental attitude come from thoughts, which is why you have to become aware of them in order not to attract unseemly circumstances, habits and beliefs and therefore an unseemly life that never helps you achieve your full potential of which you know you have a lot of.

The average human being has between 6,000–70,000 thoughts per day. Since some of these thoughts are fleeting, what we can only call "musings of the mind," thoughts are not equal. The most powerful thoughts, the ones that have the ability to change your life, are those you attach the most emotional power to and think of frequently.

Thought awareness is a learned habit that asks you to learn how to balance between obsessively monitoring all your thoughts, including fleeting ones that have a minimal effect on your life, and awareness of your most habitual thoughts.

Thought awareness is not obsessing over every thought; it's the awareness of your habitual thoughts because, as we said, only the thoughts you repeat and attach emotions to have the ability to change your life. By learning to recognize and adjust these thoughts appropriately, you can use curated thoughts (affirmations) to change any perspective and aspect of your life or circumstances.

A large percentage of our thoughts are habitual. Science estimates that because of the vast number of thoughts the human mind experiences every day, 95% of our thoughts and behaviors are automatic.

Because the mind is a professional automation machine—it automates itself to save brainpower—without thought awareness, it's possible to create a reality that is very different from the one you desire. For example, if you want a new job or a new house but your most common thoughts or beliefs towards that are negative, or you consider yourself undeserving of these things, your circumstances will change only after you change your thoughts and therefore beliefs and habits.

Affirmations for Improved Self-Image

Poor self-image (or body image) develops out of hate for oneself. At its very heart, a poor self-image is a symptom of self-hate. Self-hate is a negative character trait that you can counter with positive affirmation geared towards improving your relationship with your body.

The following affirmations will help with exactly that. As stated, and illustrated earlier, you can create self-image affirmations that stir your emotions and lead you to believe in your present awesomeness.

- "I am beautifully and wonderfully created."
- "I am perfect just as I am right now."
- "I am an attractive person who attracts positive people and creates favorable circumstances in my life."
- "I always look and feel great."
- "My body is on a temple on which I pour love, care, and affection."
- "I am a confident person admired by many."
- "I am a strong a capable person. I can overcome anything life throws at me."
- "Each moment of each day is an opportunity for self-love and care."
- "I embrace my faults."
- "I am deserving of love."
- "I believe in myself and my abilities."

- "I am very proud of the person I am right now and the person I am becoming."
- "I deserve happiness and success."
- "I always do my best."
- "I am a change catalyst. I adapt well to change."
- "I see negative criticism for what it is: one person's opinion."
- "I accept and love myself as I am right now."
- "My imperfections are what make me unique and one of a kind."
- "I treat everyone with love and kindness and everyone reciprocates in kind."
- "I let go of all negative thoughts about my body, my abilities, and accept positivity as my destiny."

A positive self-image leads to improved confidence. With that said, you can also create affirmations specifically meant to improve your confidence.

CHAPTER 10:

Choose the Words Well With Play and Creativity

Everyone has days when they don't want to do anything. You wake up and you are feeling so sluggish, unmotivated, and uninspired that you can't think of any reason why you should get out of bed. But there is one thing that anyone who ever wants to accomplish anything has in common: they get up and do it anyway.

If you want to accomplish something, then you need to get up and do it. You need to say positive things to yourself so that you can get out of bed in the morning. You need to say affirmations like "I am a smart and hardworking individual," "I am a confident person," "Today I will succeed no matter what," "Today is the day that I will finally achieve my goal of becoming a full-time writer."

Practicing the art of affirmations will not only help you with your goal but will also help in other aspects of your life. For instance, when you are feeling tired, it can actually be a good idea to practice saying affirmations to yourself. You see, there is a process that you can go through which will help fill up your brain with good thinking instead of bad ones.

- "I'm good at solving problems."
- "I have great communication skills."
- "I can motivate others through my words alone."
- "I'm an extremely loyal friend."

- "I'm a good listener."
- "I'm flexible in my thinking."
- "I often make people laugh or smile with my sense of humor."
- "People feel good around me and are happy to be in my company because they know I will support them and their ideas no matter what they are, making them feel more confident about themselves and their abilities."
- "I have extremely high standards and I'm able to meet them regularly."
- "I'm known for being generous."
- "I have intelligence, which is why I'm so good at problem-solving."
- "I'm a people lover (and people love me too!)."
- "People often admire my maturity and wisdom."
- "I have great patience and compassion for others because of my high self-esteem and self-confidence."
- "I'm a great friend."
- "I can have interesting conversations with anyone so that I never run out of things to say and always make people feel better about themselves."
- "I have a rare ability to make others laugh with my sense of humor, which is why people enjoy being in my company so much and love me for it."
- "People seem to like me even when we first meet because I am such a good listener.
- "My personality is a positive one."
- "I can read other people's feelings and needs perfectly so I know what to say and do to make them feel better about themselves, which makes them feel more comfortable around me and more confident in their decision-making abilities."

Assignment: Listen

Put on your detective cap and start listening to your words and the words of those around you. Are you noticing any patterns? Are there some changes that you wish to make to your daily vocabulary? Start connecting the dots on how your words are affecting your weight and keep recording your insights!

Change the Daily Phrases

Changing some simple daily phrases can help you change your mindset. Simply saying, "I don't want it," instead of, "I can't have it," is empowering. Here are some other suggested changes:

Instead of Saying:	Try Saying:
I will never eat this food.	I will not eat this food today.
I can't have it.	I don't want it.
I don't have time for breakfast.	I don't make time for breakfast.
I hate going to the gym.	I can move my body all day.
I messed up, so why bother?	I messed up, but I can recover.
I have no self-control.	I don't understand my triggers.

Positive Thinking Is Healthy

Most people who practice positive thinking extensively tend to experience a variety of health benefits. The thing is, there isn't too much evidence regarding the relationship between positive thinking and how it can improve your health. Studies have yet to exhibit the efficacy of positive thinking on a person's physical health.

That being said, it still is noticeable that those people who are positive experience some of the following health benefits:

- Reduced stress levels
- Better resistance to the common cold
- An increased lifespan
- Lower chance of depression
- Improved psychological health.
- Improved physical well-being.

Increase the ability to cope with situations of extreme stress.

People who think positively while continuing to have a positive outlook on life may be better equipped to handle any sort of challenge that they may encounter in life. These people approach stressful situations differently and in a way that isn't as stressful on the body. This continuous relief of stress by merely having a positive outlook on life could be one of the reasons why these people enjoy certain health benefits.

It's also a possibility that these positive people may indeed live much healthier lifestyles due to their positive outlook on life. They eat healthy food, exercise regularly, and get enough sleep. These positive thinkers also refrain from consuming alcohol and cigarettes because they know that these are things that can seriously harm your body and mind.

In short, if you continue to adopt a positive lifestyle through positive thinking, you will always try to do things that have a positive effect on your life, be it psychological or physical. Supporting others that are less fortunate than you, while keeping up with those early morning runs can help make you feel "whole" as you are doing your part for your community, as well as challenging your fitness when you are running.

Remaining Focused on Positive Thinking

In general, our thoughts will be either positive or negative (as mentioned earlier). Positive thinkers are optimists, and negative thinkers are pessimists. If you want to have a positive perspective on life, then you should (as a starting point) consider increasing your positive thoughts while decreasing your negative thoughts. One effective way of doing this is to convert your negative thinking into positive thinking.

Changing the way, you think isn't easy at all and can take time to get right. With practice, you will be able to develop new habits just by turning your negative thoughts into positive ones. Here are a few things that you can do when getting started with developing a positive outlook.

Figure Out What Needs to Be Changed

No one is perfect. We all have some form of negative trait or behavior. In most cases, these are the areas of your life that you are most likely to think about negatively. Some examples can be work, a relationship, or even a particular television show. What's the point of being negative about work when you know you will continue to work there? Why not develop a positive mindset towards work?

Some of us have constant negative thoughts related to the person we are in a relationship with. In most cases, whether the thoughts are true or not, it certainly isn't necessary and can only make you bitter towards that person. Substituting these negative thoughts of your friend or loved one for positive thoughts can undoubtedly help you improve your relationship with that person.

Trying to figure out which thoughts are negative can be difficult for most people. If you do something that makes you feel good, yet it is wrong, then how do you know if this is a negative thought or a positive one? An example is treating people unfairly or going out and overspending or overindulging. These might be things that seem ok at the time, but these are things that can have consequences at a later stage.

Take a closer look at the various aspects of your life and analyze them one by one to figure out which ones come from positive or negative thoughts. You don't have to sit down and completely re-evaluate your entire life. You can just focus on one area of your life at a time and slowly try to instill some positivity into those areas.

Keep Checking In

It's easy to fall back into the habit of thinking negatively, even after you have just decided on which of those negative thoughts you are going to replace with positive ones. With the hopes of not relapsing back to your old ways, it's best to keep on checking in on yourself periodically to analyze your progress.

You should already be very aware of the negative thoughts that you are trying to avoid. So, keeping an eye on those negative thoughts won't be difficult at all. If you find that those thoughts keep popping up, then keep trying to find a way to influence those thoughts positively. Your negative thoughts are habitual now so it will take time for you to forget them.

Stay Healthy

Exercise can definitely elevate your mood. It is also a great way to reduce stress. If you do manage to reduce your stress levels, while positively enhancing your mood, you will be setting yourself up for positive thinking. It is easier for you to think about positive things when you are in a good mood.

When it comes to exercise, you don't have to commit to an hour a day of intense workouts at the gym. Half an hour a day at home doing light exercise is sufficient. Keep at it, and you will find that you will over time develop a healthy and positive mental attitude while becoming physically fit.

Hang Out With Other Positive People

Try to hang around other people in your life that are positive and supportive of you. These are the sort of people that you can depend on when it comes to real advice and influence. In most cases, negative people will leave you feeling more stressed. If someone said something bad about you, a negative person would insist that you go and say something bad back to that person. Positive people don't entertain such behavior.

As mentioned earlier, positive people live healthy lives and have good traits. If you are constantly with a person that lives this way, you will end up living your life the same way they do. Positive people help their communities, exercise often, and are continually reading or learning something new. Spending enough time with these people will allow you the opportunity to convince yourself to adopt some of these traits.

Keep on Practicing

Continue to replace your negative thoughts with positive ones. It takes time to develop a habit (30 days). If you keep up what you are doing, then you will be able to force yourself into a complete lifestyle change. Try to find subtle and clever ways to keep yourself in check by being gentle with yourself and others. Keep encouraging yourself to think positively by making use of affirmations.

Positive Thinking and Motivation

Motivation is the reason why we engage in specific behaviors. If we do something successfully regularly, then we are most likely motivated enough to continue that action. On the other hand, if we are not really motivated to do something, then we most likely do not feel like doing anything because there is no solid reason or purpose behind our efforts.

Our fears and doubts can also cast a shadow over the reasons behind the things we do. Being genuinely motivated while remaining positive can help to keep you busy with the task at hand. You may even have the strength to take on almost any challenge that may come along.

CHAPTER 11:

Recover Your Food Instincts With Intuitive Nutrition

Intuitive eating isn't intended for weight reduction. Sadly, there might be dietitians, mentors, and different experts that sell intuitive eating as a diet, which runs counter to the thought altogether. The objective of intuitive eating is to improve your association with food. This incorporates building more beneficial food practices and trying not to control the scale. That being stated, pretty much everyone experiencing the way toward figuring out how to be an intuitive eater needs to get thinner—else, they'd as of now be intuitive eaters!

Intuitive eating enables your body to break the diet cycle and sink into its regular set point weight territory. This might be lower, higher, or a similar weight you are at present.

How Intuitive Eating Plays a Role in Healthy Living and Shopping Lifestyle

Intuitive eating guides our lives inside and out. It creates such a lot of opportunity and straightforwardness by not stressing over what I will eat or when I will eat it. I stream with what my body guides me to eat, and when it guides me to it eat— and with that, it creates opportunity inside my relationship in my body and how I feel about myself. I am more advantageous and more adjusted than I have ever been in my body and I can say that I love my body and this vessel that I am carrying on with this life in. This move-in my association with my body, food, and my general surroundings is an immediate consequence of my otherworldly voyage.

The most significant thing is to not stress over the 'right' or 'wrong' choice, and instead to distinguish how you are feeling and where in your body you think it—with the goal that you aren't eating to keep away from or conceal feelings. That way, you're eating decisions are simpler to make since they aren't enveloped with your passing feelings.

There is such a lot of opportunity and facilitate that shows up when you interface with and pursue your instinct. Shopping for food turns out to be, to a lesser degree a task or a problem and increasingly an action of happiness and articulation. To have the option to purchase what looks, sounds, and scents great (offers to the faculties) and to believe my instinct as far as what I will cook and create each day/week. It additionally makes the creation procedure progressively fun since you don't feel adhered to pursue a formula or dinner plan. Once more, there is an opportunity. Shopping for food is only an expansion of that and part of the creation procedure (where motivation comes in).

Indeed, there might, in any case, be times when you don't feel like shopping for food or preparing; however, in those minutes, you aren't hung up on it. The dread of settling on an inappropriate choice or eating inappropriate food vanishes. Intuitive eating isn't about control and dread it is about the stream and following what feels better (from a space of instinct, not damage or self-hurt).

You are beginning the adventure of understanding what foods reverberate with your body, and what doesn't-interfaces with the act of enthusiastic mindfulness. On the off chance that we shut ourselves off from feeling our feelings, at that point, we are additionally closing down our capacity to feel different sensations. Consider it like this-your body is sending you the flag of what feels better and what doesn't; however, you have unplugged the wire association between the inclination, and you are accepting and being informed of the disposition.

Having an essential comprehension of sustenance is a great spot to begin to start to teach oneself and acclimate oneself with specific establishments of pure sciences. From that point, it truly is an act of backing off and carrying your attention to how you feel, during, and after eating. At whatever point you notice examples of side effects, you should investigate. What musings did you see, how could you feel, what was going on around then? A great deal of our food and eating practices/designs have been adapted and created quite a while prior and require bringing our cognizance again into that space to develop progressive movements. The most significant piece of this procedure is to curry sympathy with you and practice non-judgment.

The diet culture is a finished square to instinct. It is established in dread and control—and expels the opportunity to interface with how you feel or what your body wants. The diet culture mirrors the longing to change and control the body, instead of helping it and work with it. It is tied in with stifling the body's direction framework (through control), which expels you further away from your instinct and the capacity to interface with your intuition through your body's informing structure. The greatest thing to perceive is that your body is profoundly insightful and realizes what to do—the more that you work with it and backing (and trust it)—the more joyful you will feel.

At whatever point we hop onto a pattern it is imperative to associate with what feels better (and to inquire as to whether this pattern genuinely impacts you or on the off chance that you are merely doing it since others are, and their outcomes entice you). A great spot to ground yourself in what your intuitive direction is, is to ask yourself "What feels useful for your spirit?"

The Health Benefits of Intuitive Eating

Improvement in Digestion

Two of the fundamental precepts of intuitive eating are to:

1. Eat just when you're ravenous
2. Eat until you're fulfilled, not stuffed

Rehearsing both of these propensities can help improve your assimilation in various manners.

- For one, eating just when you're genuinely hungry gives your stomach time to discharge your stomach from your last supper. This may appear no major ordeal, and however, when you continue eating each couple of hours and not enabling your food to process, your framework can undoubtedly move toward becoming exhausted. Your stomach needs to consistently siphon out chemicals and acids to help digest your food, while your liver is ceaselessly being attempted to channel poisons and condensation fat.
- Additionally, eating until you're full at each feast can shield your assimilation from running comfortably. You're basically "Backing up" your framework by pouring undigested food over half-processed food,

which may make you experience acid reflux, stoppage, or any number of stomach-related issues.

- Rehearsing body mindfulness, eating just until you're fulfilled, and not eating between suppers except if you're eager gives your stomach-related framework a rest with the goal that it's completely prepared to deal with your dinner.

There Is No Room for Stress

Studies have demonstrated that intuitive eaters not just appreciate a more lovely enthusiastic state than dieters, yet additionally experience enhancements in despair, nervousness, negative self-talk, and general mental prosperity when they change to eating intuitively.

The explanation behind this decrease in pressure may originate from the way that when you eat intuitively, you get the chance to concentrate more on making the most of your food as opposed to dissecting it. You additionally remove yourself from the outlook of, "I can't have that since I have to get thinner," or "I can't have carbs because I'm fat."

These sorts of responses to food put a heap of weight at the forefront of your thoughts and body, so it's no big surprise you feel better when you let them go!

A Possibility to Aid Weight Loss

Studies have likewise indicated that intuitive eaters have lower weight records (BMIs) than dieters. One of the significant purposes behind this could be because of the way that intuitive cating is anything, but difficult to adhere to (not at all like trend diets) which can prompt long haul weight reduction.

At the point when you eat intuitively, you additionally figure out how to regard the satiety flag that discloses to you when you're fulfilled, versus only eating for eating. This outcome in a natural, ideal calorie balance that could prompt weight reduction on the off chance that you've been overeating by disregarding yearning signs.

The way that intuitive eating lessens feelings of anxiety can likewise assume a job since a lot of the pressure hormone cortisol can cause fat addition.

High Self-Esteem

Notwithstanding improving eating examples and nervousness levels, contemplates have additionally demonstrated that rehearsing intuitive eating develops confidence.

For example, members in a single report experienced more acknowledgments of their bodies and less mental pain concerning their bodies. They were additionally ready to relinquish "Unfortunate weight control practices."

By improving your confidence, it's just typical that different parts of your life will improve too. At the point when you're concentrating less on not being "Sufficient," and more on tolerating yourself, you'll generally encounter less nervousness and have an increasingly inspirational point of view. Thus, this can prompt many open doors at work and enhancements in your connections.

A Decent Improvement in Body Awareness

Monitoring your body and what it's motioning to you is critical with regards to keeping up your wellbeing. On the off chance that you listen intently, your body will offer you inconspicuous hints that something isn't right, enabling you to give it what it needs before it turns into a significant issue.

Take, for instance, indications of supplement inadequacies. Numerous individuals are so separated from their bodies that they don't see unobtrusive signs of supplement insufficiency, similar to an absence of vitality or shivering in their grasp and feet. When they do understand, the inadequacy has turned out to be dangerous to such an extent that they need to go to the specialist to get it dealt with.

Intuitive eating is tied in with connecting with your body's sign of craving and satiety. Be that as it may, when you start focusing on these signs, you'll begin to be hyper-mindful of different signs your body is emitting. This will enable you to be in line with what you need consistently, so you can deal with it before it turns into an all-out issue.

CHAPTER 12:

Learn to Say "No" to Those Who Want to Limit and Want to Change You

Negative people can be a drag on your weight-loss journey. If you feel like you're fighting a losing battle with the temptation of tasty, fattening treats, it can be really easy to give up and wallow in self-pity. Weight is often meant as an external marker of your worth, so if someone criticizes or judges you for your body or weight-loss efforts, it's easy to internalize those negative feelings and retreat back into comfort foods that make your waistline grow.

But there's a difference between negative people and negative situations. Negative people are highly problematic. Their negativity can affect your weight-loss results for the worse, but low self-esteem rarely causes weight gain. In fact, contrary to popular belief, rejection by others does not cause negative emotions to "feed" into body weight gain. Also, if you engage in healthy behaviors, people will generally accept and appreciate your healthier choices. So, what do you do when a negative person is bugging you? How can you deal with the negativity without giving up on your weight-loss goals? Here are some ideas for adapting to the negativity that keeps you from succeeding:

Learn to Say "No" and Create Some Distance

Perhaps it's easiest to befriend a negative person who's giving you grief. This will make it easier to avoid the person and the negative conversations. Try to avoid listening to someone's constant talk of self-hatred or guilt. These people are gloomy and you'll start taking on their negativity. It's like a virus that will make you sick!

Instead, hang out with positive people who are healthier than you. You'll be motivated by them. These people will help build your confidence and keep you inspired in your weight-loss efforts.

We all know that saying "yes" is important. It's part of the foundation upon which we build our relationships with others, it's something that keeps us from getting overwhelmed by commitments, and it also makes things more interesting when we have a tight schedule! But saying "yes" to everything isn't always the best way to proceed. A person can get stuck in a rut of being so busy doing for others that they don't have time for themselves. Or they might feel like it's their responsibility to take on more than they can handle because of an expectation from others or from themselves. Sometimes, we rush through the day and make commitments that we don't have the time to meet. And it's not just our work commitments that might take up more than we want. Family and friends might place expectations on us, or we might put expectations on ourselves.

Perhaps you've heard the phrase that goes like this: "If you don't say 'no' to someone, they'll say 'yes' to you." This means that if you don't take care of yourself first and let others know what works for you, they'll push their own agenda onto your schedule. And this can cause several worries for you! But it doesn't have to be this way. You can master how to say "no" in a way that will also help you become more organized.

The key to saying "no" is being clear about what you're trying to accomplish. That means giving yourself time to do things for yourself in a way that will support your best interests. These are important tasks that you can't just let slide and ignore. We all have those things that we want to do every day, which adds up over time. You may opt to go for a walk, read a book, or meditate. You might also want to clean out your closets, organize your filing system, or take care of other personal matters. If you don't make time for these every day, you'll end up feeling frustrated with yourself. You'll feel like you aren't accomplishing much, and there's no way that you can meet everyone's expectations all the time! So, if your agenda is so tight that you're always in a hurry, it's important to find a chance for the things that are essential to you.

You might also want to think about how you view your commitments. Are you setting yourself up for failure by making commitments that don't end up in your calendar? You might have committed to a friend only to find out that he's not available, or you might have been planning on meeting another set of friends but ended up having to cancel everything because of an unexpected work obligation. Sometimes these things happen and you need to let others know that you can't meet their expectations.

Don't get stuck feeling guilty for saying "no. "One of the best ways to be able to say "no" is to have a very precise comprehension of what you can and cannot do. If you don't have this understanding, your tendency will be toward saying "yes" or giving in to other people. But you mustn't do this! Having a realistic view of what's going on with your commitments will ensure that you won't feel like a failure if you need to say no for reasons beyond your control.

One way to summarize this is by saying "no" in a way that will support your best interests. You're going to have some things that you can't make happen, so you need to know what those are. You may discover that you don't want to do certain things for yourself. Or maybe you have a home and family that needs attention, and that's something you feel like you have to prioritize. You must know when it's appropriate to say "yes" and when it's time to say "no." You'll feel much more fulfilled if you do this, and you won't have so many of your days feeling like they were wasted with things that didn't matter.

Positive Behaviors

Indeed, rejection doesn't cause body weight gain (despite what we've been told). But it's easy to take rejection personally and let it affect your mood and habits. You might feel inadequate and want to retreat into your old comfort eating habits. The thing is, that if you feel better about yourself, you'll be more open to criticism or rejection by others.

When you feel confident in yourself, you'll be open to new opportunities. You won't be self-conscious about what people will say about your weight-loss efforts because you won't focus on weight as a measure of your worth. If you need some motivation to stay the course, focus on the positive behaviors that will leave people impressed and not critical of your weight loss.

If you're trying to grow, it's not uncommon to encounter people who are unaware of or opposed to, your growth. These people may be toxic; they may have development goals that don't align with yours. They may disrupt your focus and cause you to lose sight of the goal...but they aren't the real problem.

The Real Problem Is Fear

That's right, fear of failure and fear of growth. These are the true reasons you're being held back. People are scared. It's the world we live in; they're scared of failure as a result of their lives. However, they can't be afraid because if they can't grow, then there's no way to fail. But failing can cause them to retreat, so protecting their ego is key to their continued survival in this world, and it provides them with a sense of security.

These people will step in to stop you from growing and may do so successfully for a while. But they're not the real enemy. The real enemy is fear; the fear of being thought of as weak or foolish for trying to grow, and the fear of looking stupid because they failed to understand your growth.

Those people who stand in your way aren't truly your enemies; they are merely obstacles that need to be overcome, just like any obstacle in life. The real enemies are the ones you've put into your heart that led you to believe that you're incapable of growing, and that fear is what's holding you back.

So, what do you do with people who stop you from growing?

The answer is simple: You stop caring about them.

If these people are blocking your growth, treat them like an obstacle and pass them by. If they're standing in your way, don't waste energy worrying about them. Don't worry; they're not investing their lives into achieving your goal. And even if they were, it doesn't matter because you're the only person who can make something happen.

There's a certain process when it comes to overcoming obstacles in life: You move forward, or you move backward. Either way, you can't waste time on what you don't want or need. That's why it's important to stop worrying about these people... because they are non-threats and not relevant to your path to growth.

There's only one person who controls your growth, and that's you. You are the one who makes it happen. You and you alone control whether you stop growing or continue moving forward. You are the one who has to decide what to do with people who threaten your growth...and nothing more than that.

Don't let fear stand in your way; never allow fear (or anyone) to hold you back from becoming everything you can become.

If you've ever worked for a difficult boss, dealt with an obsessive ex, or simply found yourself the target of someone who is overly needy and passive-aggressive, then you know how hard our society can be on people who say no. Telling others "no" isn't as simple as it might seem if you have to appease their constant demands for your time and energy in exchange for their silence or compliance. It can take a lot of practice and patience before the word becomes more natural to us.

When you work with, live with, or are related to a person who is manipulative or passive-aggressive, it is difficult to refuse their demands. Instead of going along with them and trying to figure out the best way to avoid saying no, learn how to say what you mean clearly and effectively. For example, if someone pressures you for more time than you can afford to give, then it's time to learn how to say no gracefully. Simply saying that you already have commitments that day is not enough in these situations. If it's okay for them to take several hours, then it's also okay for you to refuse to give them more time.

On the other hand, if someone tries to avoid taking responsibility for a decision or agreement with you, then learning how to say no gracefully might backfire on them. There are so many ways that people can get around others when they are trying to avoid making their own commitments and decisions clear. This is when you have to learn how to say no without saying no. After all, it's never a good idea to confront manipulative or passive-aggressive people directly if it can be avoided.

CHAPTER 13:

"No" to Imposed Duties and Obligations

Duties imposed on you by others often make you resentful and resentful people have a harder time staying productive. Duties are considered burdens and some duties can only be fulfilled if you get angry, or neglect your self-care, or go out of your comfort zone. It's important to set boundaries with the people around us. Learn how to say no in healthy ways that maintain good relationships with those around you.

Saying no when you feel it is not only the right thing to do, but it is also the best for your self-esteem. It can be hard, however, to say no. It may seem like you're being disrespectful or uncooperative if you turn others down when they ask for help or favors.

You may be afraid that if you don't say yes to everything that people will think of you as selfish and uncaring. But saying no is a sign of maturity and can help you keep your dignity intact. Each time you say no, you are practicing independence and standing up for your rights. It takes courage to say no, but it will also take courage to stick to your guns if someone accuses you of being selfish or narcissistic.

Say "No" in a Way That Supports Your Self-Esteem

One way to lessen the sting of saying no is not only to be firm in doing so but also to explain why. For instance, you can tell the person asking you to do a favor that you would like to but have too many commitments at the moment. Or you can tell them that you need to concentrate on work right now and can't help out. Knowingly, it is simpler said than done, but it is a good idea.

When you are clear about why you are saying no, your self-esteem will be enhanced because when someone asks for your help and true to your word, you will say no without being disrespectful or rude.

When you say no to people, you ultimately come across as a person who is strong and independent. You can say no without feeling bad about it, or without giving the impression that you are unappreciative. You can also be nice to people when they ask for your help, and you should be nice to them.

As long as you are polite while saying no, it is a healthy way of handling things.

For example, if someone asks you to take care of their pet, you can say no and tell the person that it is a responsibility that you are not ready to fulfill at this time. You can also add on a polite statement of your appreciation for their kindness.

You also don't have to let people down face-to-face. You can say no in a post. If you have to say something, you can use these helpful phrases:

"I do hope that I get a chance to help out and would seriously enjoy it. However, I would like to be able to focus on my own projects this month and next month, and I don't think this is feasible right now."

You don't have to let them down in person or verbally, but your word is really important. Be positive and get to say no without feeling bad or angry.

Saying no is not rude. You have the right to say no. So don't be intimidated by people who want you to give up something for them that you need for yourself, such as your free time or your energy.

Your task today is to learn how to say no in a way that supports your self-esteem. Say no to people in a way that lets them know you understand their need for your help or your time, but that you also have needs of your own.

- **Step 1:** Start by saying "no" to a few things today that are not good for you.
- **Step 2:** Look at how it feels to say no and compare the feeling of being uncooperative with what it means to be responsible for yourself.
- **Step 3:** When possible, say no in a face-to-face situation.
- **Step 4:** Analyze how you feel about what you are saying no to.
- **Step 5:** If saying no is difficult, try to do it in a nice way that doesn't send an unkind message.
- **Step 6:** Remember that you are saying no for your good.
- **Step 7:** Don't worry about being uncooperative or selfish; being responsible for yourself is much more important than pleasing everyone around you.
- **Step 8:** Be clear about what you want.
- **Step 9:** Practice being nice to people while you are saying no.

- **Step 10:** Just say no and don't give reasons unless asked for them.
- **Step 11:** If you can't say no, be absent. You do not have to be available all the time.
- **Step 12:** Keep track of whether or not your "no" is working well for your self-esteem and your stress level.

I know how difficult it is to say no. But if you keep in mind that you are being responsible for yourself, you will eventually say no without feeling guilty.

Remember that saying no isn't selfish or uncaring. Rather, it is an act of self-responsibility that helps to lower your stress level, which in turn can help you get a handle on your quality of life.

Saying no will also help you keep your word longer. If you really want to say no, it will be easier for you to do so because you will be more self-aware and mindful.

When you are clear about why you say "no," your self-esteem will be enhanced because when someone asks for your help and true to your word, you will say no without being disrespectful or rude.

When you say no to people, you ultimately come across as a person who is strong and independent. You are capable of taking care of yourself and your needs, and you don't allow other people to interfere with your goals.

Learning how to say no is often a matter of practice. You have to get used to saying "no" for the first time before you can easily say it when it counts for you.

Make time for a few hours during the day tomorrow to practice saying no in several different ways. If you want to practice with your friends, say no in a way that doesn't make them feel bad or rejected.

Try to do at least three different things during the day that require you to say no to something or someone.

For example, if someone asks you for something and it's not good for you, then tell them "no" without making the person feel angry or rejected. Alternatively, if you are in a situation where you need to decline something that someone else is offering, then say "no" in a nice way without being underhanded or rude.

You may have to repeat some exercises a few times before you get it right, but just keep practicing until you feel confident in your ability to say no.

Another way of saying no and still being polite or nice is to "save face" with the other person. This means that you can say "no" and then still show them that you respect their opinion and feelings by telling them that you will have a better time doing something else.

Example:

"I really appreciate your offer to help, but I would like to do something else this evening. Thank you so much for the offer to hang out, but I am going to meet up with my friends instead."

The basic idea is that you are saying no and saving face. You are still saying no, but you can also let the person know that you respect them without making them feel rejected or unwanted.

Decide on a "No" Strategy—Pick One and Stick to It

Deciding on an assertive no strategy will help you say no in a consistent way. This strategy should work in any situation where someone is asking you for something.

The "Magic Object" Strategy

This strategy is simple and effective. The idea behind it is that you take an object (could be anything from a pencil to a book) and hold it out to the person. When they ask you for something, instead of saying "no," just hand them your magic object. Then when they ask why to explain that the object you are holding is all the time that they get.

This is a great strategy to use when you don't want to or are unable to be rude. It lets the person know that you simply don't have the time, but it also doesn't offend them.

The "Drop an Object" Strategy

This is another strategy for when you need to turn down an invitation. This one works best in social settings.

When you are being invited out, but you don't want to go with the person asking, drop an object.

The object can be anything small like a business card or your keys. You can even pretend to have an item fall from your pocket or bag when they offer to walk you there.

If this doesn't get the point across, just tell them that you suddenly remembered something really important and have to leave immediately.

The "Best Friend" Strategy

This strategy works best when you have to turn down an invitation for an entire evening. Use this one whenever you want to say no without offending anyone.

Say that you would love to go out with them sometime but can't do so that night because your best friend just canceled on you and begged for your company. Tell them that you'll call them later in the week and catch up with them then.

The "Alibi" Strategy

If you don't feel comfortable saying no to someone, simply tell them that you're not available that day or at that time. If they ask why just shrug your shoulders and say that something else came up.

This strategy is especially useful when you are asked to do something last minute. You can just say that you already have plans at that time.

The "Respect" Strategy

If someone is looking for an excuse and is not taking your "no," you can try telling them that it isn't respectful of them to ask. Tell them that you respect their wishes but don't feel comfortable doing something they want you to do.

This strategy is effective in many situations. You can use it to turn down an invitation, refuse to do a favor, say no to someone's request for money or time, and even say no to anything that you don't want to do.

The "Reputation" Strategy

If you are asked by someone how they can get a good reputation, you can give them this advice. Tell them that by helping them, they will earn a reputation while supporting their goals.

Remember that when someone asks you for help and you really want to say no, just don't give any excuses. Sometimes, the most honorable way out is just telling someone that you cannot help them or support what they are doing.

CHAPTER 14:

Take Care of Yourself

What does your body tell you in your life about the need to heal the wound? Every day, the body sends out signals which let you know how safe it really is in general. Aches and pains are usually a warning somewhere deep inside that something is wrong. Some of the origins are a little more obvious than others. It is up to you to take the time to listen to the hints about your overall health that your body offers so that you have an idea of how you can take care of yourself. Here are some ways to do so:

Think Positive Thoughts

Nearly every religion in the world states that positive thinking plays a significant role in healing. When you have to heal the body, it is a good idea to spend a little time thinking positively each day. You may just find that in this age-old philosophy, you have made a believer out of yourself in no time when you start to experience the power of positive thinking working inside your body to build a healthier you.

Exercise

Exercise is one of the most overlooked factors in healing the body. Over the years, it has been reduced to a fitness role and is equated with the need to keep in shape or assist in that goal rather than a balanced practice in and of itself. Exercise releases endorphins to provide relief from pain and a sense of happiness and well-being at large.

Good Diet

A balanced diet is a wonderful resource for healing your body as much as it can cause you to know it. To maintain maximum health, you need other nutrients. Unfortunately, we are in a world consumed with fast-food chains, and very few people get the nutrients required for optimum health. That's why it's important to bear in mind other choices like vitamin supplements—although they're not nearly as successful as getting the nutrients through your diet.

Adopt Healthy Habits

There are some actions that you can utilize that will facilitate improved health. Replace antibacterial soap with your regular hand soap. Often wash your hands and wash them well. Teach your family how to wash their faces, cover their mouths, and use sanitizing hand wipes or liquid cleaners in public to reduce the risk of taking home infections and diseases. Such practices can seem too simplistic but may result in prevention, which is often the best treatment, allowing the body to heal.

Protecting the Body With Hypnosis

Self-hypnosis is just another means of protecting the body from illnesses of all kinds. Many ways mastering the art of self-hypnosis can help in your struggle, whether you are trying to reject cancer that is just as hard to take over or ward off the common cold.

Hypnosis can help you relax, open your mind to positive thinking, help the nutrients get where they are best served, and help boost immunity, among other great things.

Take Control of Your Healing Process

It is time for you to take control of your body and its process of healing. Whether you are using one or all of the above techniques, if you listen to your body and react accordingly—for the best possible health outcome—you can find real help when it comes to healing the body.

Hypnosis is a powerful mode that can help your body stop unwanted habits and then start to heal and rejuvenate your body. It's all about the computer device situated within the brain.

Stress will show itself in all different kinds of scenarios... Ranging from being depressed to violent. Contrary to common opinion, medications just exacerbate the condition while making huge bucks for the pharmaceuticals. Seek your nearest hypnotherapist first before you go to get medication to be healthy again. You're going to be happier faster, and it's going to last a lot longer!

Will they hypnotize you? Hey! The condition you strive to achieve is one of absolute relaxation as though you're about to fall asleep. You are still very much in charge because we are enhancing your drive to do what you set out to do.

Hypnosis is initially a type of deep relaxation that allows the client to take an imagined journey. The imagination is where you build a new, vibrant vision for what you want to be like in your future.

When your critical mind is in a very deep relaxed state, it calms down from that constant thinking that says: "I can't just leave," or "It's just too hard to quit." Side-stepping the critical mind lets you become motivated to accomplish what you felt was impossible before. Not only does it work well with smoking, but it also works well in sports, handling discomfort, and even taking exams.

Old habits of thinking can be replaced quickly and lovingly with fresh, wonderful optimistic thoughts that can make leaving such a positive force in your life. Only imagine if you can avoid obsessing about a question, you can actually do something, be, have anything. You broke the habit, and you can achieve anything set out to do. Your level of confidence goes sky-high!

Hypnotherapy will help move the body into new wellness. Your cells can be ordered to heal through the science of Epigenetics. Hypnosis is the best way to help cancer patients help the body cure at faster speeds, particularly with surgeries. Studies that show hypnosis heals the body have been performed to minimize bleeding, swelling, and bruises, as well as speed up the recovery process 10 times faster. In addition to that, it has been established that 10 minutes of hypnosis actually reduce blood pressure and lower cholesterol. If you want to quit smoking, eradicate a phobia, help heal cancer or pain, then just use your strong and focused mind to seek it out without medication. It is a lot easier than you could ever imagine. You become a champion, and you'll be shocked by how strong you are.

Get Clear on What You Want

It is through your dreams and desires that you develop and advance. You are an everlasting being and will perpetually have desires. It is a critical component in the development of life; yours, yet besides, the Universe. Without desire, you can't develop and would stop existing. Your dreams and desires may happen as intended at the end alone without deliberate aim; however, why leave it to risk when you can manifest what you need all the more rapidly? This is the place clarity comes in. Getting clear and focusing on precisely what you need to create in your life accelerates the process.

Think about every one of the accompanying aspects of your life and compose a rundown of what you need:

- **Your values:** What is most important to you—achievement, opportunity, satisfaction? Identifying your values will assist you with getting clear on the essence of what you need and will fill in as the establishment for your dream life. If you don't have the experience you need, you are most likely living from a different arrangement of values than is required for what you need. Consider reprioritizing your top benefits to make a higher amount of what you generally need.

- **Ideal self:** Identifying the qualities of your perfect self will assist you with reclaiming your true identity and adjust you to the individual you were born to be.

- **Well-being and body:** What are your ideal for your wellbeing and body? What amount do you gauge? What sorts of nourishments do you eat? Do you work out? If things being what they are, how and how frequently, how would you feel physically? What do you resemble?

- **Money-related abundance:** What does your ideal budgetary circumstance resemble? What amount of cash do you make? What are your wellsprings of pay? What amount of money do you have in your bank account? Do you contribute?

- **Profession:** What is your ideal work circumstance? Do you work with others or alone? Is it accurate to say that you are your supervisor, perhaps a businessperson? What exercises would you say you are doing? What abilities do you use?

- **Personal relationship:** Think about your ideal cozy relationship. How can it look and feel? What does your sweetheart resemble? What character attributes does he/she have? What sorts of things do you do together? How would you feel when you're with him/her?

- **Different relationships:** What does your ideal relationship with others (relatives, companions, colleagues) resemble? How would you feel in these relationships?

- **Home environment:** Where do you live? Who do you live with? What sort of house do you have? What number of rooms and restrooms? How would you feel at home?

- **Profound life:** What are your supernatural beliefs? What exercises do you do (meditation, go to chapel, and so on.)?

- **Fun and recreation:** What exercises do you accomplish for the sake of entertainment? Where are you? Who is with you?

Include or change things as you consider them: After some time, your vision will turn out to be increasingly clearer until, in the end, your life will start to unfurl as you have depicted.

CHAPTER 15:

Express Your Feelings Fearlessly

We all struggle with the fear of being judged when expressing our feelings. There is a stigma about sharing vulnerable feelings and emotions that are often not considered valid. You may feel like you have to hold back your feelings, avoid discussing them or even bottle them up inside. Ultimately, your negative emotions could lead to a toxic cycle that negatively affects your physical and mental health as well as overall mental well-being.

Feelings are important to our overall well-being. They may be considered an emotion, but they support the energy and flow of life. If you are able to express your feelings openly and honestly, they may lead to more feeling-centered relationships, as well as a deeper connection with yourself. Ultimately this can create a better understanding of yourself while reducing conflicts in relationships.

Fears of Expressing Feelings

We have some fears about expressing what we feel. We are afraid of the way others may react when we are open to discuss our feelings. We may be concerned they won't listen and they will judge us for feeling the way we do. These concerns lead us to avoid sharing our feelings so that they can't be criticized or judged. As a result, these worries or fears can lead to stress, anxiety, and even depression.

We all have fears of expressing our feelings. We might fear telling our parents that we love them for not being able to handle it or be afraid of what others will think about us if we openly show our opinions on a subject. As human beings, we need a way to express ourselves to feel complete and whole. Without expression, any event in life can leave us feeling unsatisfied and lost.

Whether it be feelings of uncertainty or anger, we all have a fear of being judged or not being accepted for what we feel. We live in an age where showing emotions such as fear, love, and sadness are commonplace. By this, I mean that crying on television shows is considered a normal form of expression. These shows are not criticized for conveying such emotions to their viewers; it is no longer strange to see a woman shed tears on a show when her boyfriend has left her.

If you have ever had a fear of expressing feelings, you know it can be stressful and difficult to deal with. It can make you avoid getting close to people or limit your self-expression.

Fear of expressing feelings can be a lifelong trait for some women, according to Algoe. This may be caused by issues related to early childhood or how they were treated during their teens. It is also possible that mothers might have hidden their feelings when their children were young and the child was unable to express them. "Sometimes women will know that they want to express their feelings but find it difficult," says Algoe.

As a result, the affected women might not fully understand the range of their feelings. This can be particularly true if they grew up in a family where self-expression is not encouraged. Women may also have trouble expressing their feelings in public, which is a particularly frequent fear for those who have stayed in families that were not emotionally expressive.

Even though they may fear expressing how they feel, most women can do so when they are with their closest friends or partners. This is because these individuals are usually accepting of and supportive of them.

What is even more astounding is how women have adapted to the world in which we live. I believe that fear of expressing feelings in women stems from society's pressures. These pressures are unavoidable, yet they can be overcome by choosing not to let them control us.

Society as a whole believes that there is an inability to express oneself without being judged negatively. This false assumption can be seen through the media, movies, and television. We see women portrayed in movies that are always crying or somehow end up in a situation where the whole scene is focused on the woman's feelings.

When watching these shows and movies, women tend to feel how they think they should feel. This is because they do not want to be known as cold-hearted or uncaring people. They are trying to connect with the characters on a deeper level by thinking about things that make them sad for them to understand what the character feels.

They want to be empathized with because they are so used to being sympathized with. This is not a bad thing, as they want to feel connected to others and not as an outcast who is different from everyone else. It is human nature, however, that women do not want to feel isolated by such feelings.

The fear of expressing feelings in women stems from the need for comfort and belonging through acceptance of these feelings. They feel as if the world will come crashing down on them if they begin to express themselves. This is why they do not show their feelings.

As a result of this feeling of isolation, women often become distant from others and focus on themselves. Focusing on themselves is a natural response to cope with the loneliness that results from expressing feelings that may be considered wrong or taboo. This distance from others prevents them from feeling these negative emotions that may be associated with the feelings they have inside of them.

However, in the end, expressing feelings of sadness is a normal way for people to release these feelings. It is a way for them to learn more about themselves and realize what they need to change in their lives. It is important that people feel the freedom to express whatever they want, as it allows them to love themselves and accept who they really are.

Women need to accept themselves. They must acknowledge that they can love themselves and never be controlled by other people's opinions or values. Women need to know that what we do and how we live our lives is our decision. These decisions are not made for us, nor should they be, as we are all free individuals in this world who make our decisions.

I believe that it is in each individual's best interests to express themselves regardless of how others react to it. By overcoming these fears, we allow others to accept us for who we are, and not for what we do or how others expect us to act. Women must realize the value of truly living their lives as an individual who is free of restrictions.

How to Overcome Fears of Expressing Feelings

If you have avoided showing your emotions, it is important to recognize that feelings can be a normal part of who you are. It is also important to remember that many people suppress their emotions to avoid upsetting others. This can lead to unhappiness and changes in how they process information.

One option for women who are worried about expressing themselves is taking social media breaks from their friends or other loved ones. "This can help you get perspective on what you are doing and how your interactions with others affect your emotions," says Algoe.

It is also important for women who fear expressing their feelings to set realistic goals for themselves. "Make a list of small goals for yourself and start working on them one at a time," she recommends. "They could be as simple as initiating a conversation with a stranger in line at the grocery store or talking to the cashier. Anxious people often find it difficult to go outside at all. They might stay inside and shut themselves off from the rest of the world. It is important to overcome these fears and gradually face them." Setting small goals helps these individuals get used to talking with others. This can lead to more self-confidence and fewer feelings of tension.

Making sure you have eaten a balanced meal can also help you feel less afraid or anxious about expressing your emotions, according to Algoe. She also recommends talking to a professional if you are having difficulty overcoming your fear of expressing how you feel.

Getting Help for the Fear of Expressing Feelings in Women

If you would like to receive help for the fear of expressing feelings in women, it is a good idea to see a psychologist with experience in this area. They can help you explore the reasons why you feel this way and how to overcome it. They can also aid with taking small steps towards being more open about how you feel.

"In cognitive behavioral therapy, you can practice saying what you are feeling," she says. "This might be challenging, but it will help you develop more confidence and show your emotions."

When it comes to seeking help for this issue, women should not be embarrassed or ashamed. They should also realize that support is available and that they will eventually be able to fully control their fear of expressing what they feel.

Meditation can be a great way to learn how to express your feelings. It can help you become more aware of your emotions and learn how to communicate in healthy ways. The first step is learning to identify what you feel emotional. You may have been taught not to talk about feelings, but you don't have to keep them bottled up inside indefinitely. Instead, start taking the step to speak out loud about what is on your mind!

Meditation can help you realize that you have the right to express your feelings and not be criticized for doing so. Once you become more aware of your emotions, you may notice that they are not as overwhelming or intense as they once were. Meditation can also help transform negative emotions into a positive outlook.

When it comes to emotional expression, it's important to be okay with being honest about how you feel. Seeing or understanding that you are worthy of expression, provides you the space to share feelings and express them. And this allows others to accept you and your emotions. As a result, you become more confident in expressing your emotions, which ultimately helps to build a healthy sense of self-esteem.

CHAPTER 16:

Find Your Femininity

Everyone has a definition of what it means to be feminine. Some might be very traditional, and others might feel like you are more "feminine" than they are. There is no one-size-fits-all response to the conundrum 'what does it mean to be feminine?' but we will explore some ideas on what being a woman means for many of them today.

What Is Femininity?

Femininity is nothing more than a feeling. It's a combination of emotions, values, and behaviors that make you feel beautiful, confident, and strong. Femininity isn't about what you look like or how much you weigh; it's about the way you feel. To be feminine means to take care of yourself, to love yourself, and to give back to the world around you.

Femininity isn't about being nice or making others feel good. It's about leading; it's about being a role model for those around you. Femininity means taking care of yourself so that you can take care of others. It means leading by example and showing people that when you are ready to commit, it doesn't mean you're not feminine enough to be in a relationship with them. It means you love yourself enough to understand that this is the right thing for you.

Femininity doesn't just mean being feminine in society's eyes. It means showing respect for yourself and those around you, whether it's your family, friends, or colleagues at work. Be honest about who you are and allow other people to see the beauty of your uniqueness. It doesn't matter what others perceive of you; it's about the way that you feel when you're around them.

The things that make us feminine might vary from person to person and can change over time. But one thing is for sure, being feminine is something you have to do for yourself.

In today's society, a female is expected to be thin and delicate. This has led to weight-loss hysteria in both men and women. The reason for this is that society's beliefs that being thin will increase femininity. A study with participants ranging from ages 18–65 suggests that this may not be the case. It was found that a majority of the participants believed that weight loss can increase femininity. In addition, the researchers concluded that for men, this may be true, but in the case of women, "feminine attractiveness was best predicted by general healthiness and waist-to-hip ratio."

Another study also suggests much the same thing. The study involved participants ranging from 18 and 60 years old. The findings showed that "participants think thin people are healthier and more attractive. They believed that thinner was better, regardless of whether the model was male or female." In the end, participants concluded that thin people were healthier and more attractive. This can be defined in several ways, but to the researchers, it means that being "slender" is a feminine trait. There is also proof that sows an increase in femininity when one loses weight.

Research implemented by the University of Toronto states, "Lose weight and you'll feel more feminine." Participants ranging in age from 18–29 concluded that being thin is more attractive. The findings of this study also suggest a correlation between femininity and weight loss. It was found that participants who lost the most weight were the most desirable. These results can also be interpreted in many ways, but to the researchers, it shows that being "feminine" is linked to weight loss. To further support this hypothesis, researchers have found that just one pound of body fat can make someone seem at least 10 years older than their actual age.

The media can influence how one looks at thinness and weight loss. A study done in hopes of determining the effects of thinness on attractiveness was conducted with Caucasian females ranging in age from 19–32. Participants were shown five different female figures that varied in body size. After each figure was shown, a questionnaire was given to the participants. This survey consisted of 25 questions that required the participants to rate the figure based on a variety of characteristics or traits including femininity and attractiveness. Based on the survey, the researchers concluded that participants' ratings of feminine attractiveness were best predicted by their perceptions of general healthiness and waist-to-hip ratio. This suggests that particular body shapes are more attractive than others.

However, not all studies suggest that losing weight can increase femininity. One experiment done at Tel Aviv University had participants look at photographs of extremely thin women. Research has shown that anorexia nervosa can be a behavior to cope with stress, depression, and anxiety. Some participants were given the task of evaluating the personality characteristics of a thin woman by looking at her photo. The majority of the participants who were shown these photos "rated the women as less lively, cheerful, energetic, confident and sociable than did a second group." This suggests that thinness does not necessarily increase femininity.

In summary, several research studies have suggested that weight loss increases femininity. One experiment done with Caucasian females ranging in age from 19–32 used 25 questions to conclude that thinness is preferred by both men and women.

Dieting is a fast-growing focus in the Western world. In recent years, with the improvement in food technology and exercise science, it has become more possible than ever to lose weight without going on a diet. Thinner people are often seen as more feminine due to their narrow waists and fuller hips. The weight they have lost however has more often than not been put on their faces or chests. Many women wish to be more feminine but still have the ability to eat whatever they want without putting any extra weight on their lower regions, which will be seen as unattractive by many males worldwide.

The word dieting comes from the French word "diété." It is a compound of "Dieu" and "été," meaning "to discipline, to train, or instruct." The English word diet is derived from the same Latin root as the French word, "diété." This word was a derivative of "diétas," which was a compound of "diere" and "idion," meaning "to assign" or "to put in place." Diets are comparable to training regimes. The aim of both is to develop and improve one's physical condition.

The many variations of the diet industry include weight-loss programs, diets for specific medical conditions, and those that are simply for aesthetic reasons. Some of these diets are so strict that they resemble training programs, not only by how they work but by the costs and time commitments involved.

The three main ways to measure attractiveness are healthiness, body fat, and weight. These three categories can be broken down even further into several separate factors. The most important factor in all three categories is a low waist-hip ratio (WHR). This is sometimes referred to as an hourglass figure. Women have a waist that is at least 70% as wide as their hips.

Waist-hip ratios are an important determinant of attractiveness, although by itself it is not a perfect measure. The waist is found by dividing the hip circumference by the circumference of the waist. Once this measurement is made, it is necessary to take some consideration for breast size. Since women's breasts do not stretch with their waists, two modifications must be made. The first is to add half of the difference in their breast size to the waist measurement. The second is to add half of the difference in their breast size to the hip measurement. With these two modifications, it can be assumed that the woman has roughly an hourglass figure and that she should have an attractive face and body for her height.

Once a woman has achieved this hourglass figure, she will want to make sure that she reduces any excess fat so that all other parts of her body are proportionate with it. The weight that a woman puts on her face and chest can make her seem bigger than she actually is, and therefore, less attractive.

This excess fat may take the form of either excess fat cells or a reduction in fat cells due to water loss. Both are undesirable as they can cause an unnatural distribution of fat in a woman's body. However, there are ways that a woman can burn these calories without losing any from around her waist. This is accomplished by engaging in regular exercise.

There are types of exercises that target specific parts of the body to burn fat deposits, such as aerobic exercises. This type of exercise will result in a loss of unwanted fat, mainly around the midsection and thighs. Examples include jogging, running, and similar activities that elevate heart rate. Although aerobic exercise is beneficial because it burns calories overall, this type of exercise is not the best way to specifically burn fat from around the hips or waist area.

Instead, women should focus on cardiovascular exercises that target fat. Examples of such exercises include running, swimming, and cycling. These types of exercise require an elevated heart rate to be exercised at the fastest possible speed without increasing the risk of injury. They will also result in greater energy expenditure in general and therefore a better way to burn calories from around the waist area. Women should make sure that they do not restrict their diet before engaging in cardiovascular exercise because it may lead to them gaining weight from overconsumption of calories.

Swimming is a particularly beneficial form of exercise because it burns both calories and fat. The activity also promotes muscle tone, which will help to reduce the appearance of cellulite, especially in the thighs. Even though swimming is more of aerobic activity, women should not restrict their diet before engaging in it because it can lead to overconsumption.

Women should also be aware of the amount of food they are consuming as well as the types of foods that they are consuming. No one diet plan will work well for all women because not all women have the same body type or genetic make-up. To determine how many calories a woman requires; she must first estimate her basal metabolic rate. This can be done by estimating the number of calories she burns at rest.

More active women may also want to add some extra calories to account for their higher activity level. Once the calorie requirement has been determined, then it is possible to determine a diet plan that will work best for her.

CHAPTER 17:

Cultivate Your Independence

When you want to start losing weight, take control of your body and lose the pounds permanently. Learn about the different ways that people can take control of their bodies to shed pounds.

Some people may think it is easier than they think, while others may find themselves limited and not sure where to begin. This will provide an overview of how a person can get started as well as some helpful tips for success. These are just some samples of what is possible when you take charge and become accountable for your physical well-being.

- If you want to control your body, you will need to start an exercise program. Everyone will have their individual explanations for choosing from the many kinds of physical activity and workouts that are available. If you cannot decide which is right for you, talk to your doctor or a fitness guru about what might work most suitable for you.
- You may also want to start changing the way you eat by choosing healthier foods in small portions along with water instead of sugary drinks and other empty calories that are less healthy options.
- Finally, it is also advised that you do some kind of bodyweight exercise. Start simple and build your level of fitness by increasing the intensity of each workout slowly over time.

Having an accountability partner can be very advantageous in the beginning, but if you can improve past that level, then an accountability partner will not be necessary. If you aim to lose pounds and keep it off, a few months or even a year later then that can work for many people as well. Whatever you decide to do, it is important to take the time to really think about what changes you need to make to achieve the body that you want.

Taking control of your body does not mean that you can never eat those foods or drinks again. You may find that a treat from time to time does not have as great an impact on your weight-loss goals as you might have expected. Always remember that if food is necessary for physical survival, it should be eaten. What it means is that you are deciding to control your body and have it work for you rather than against you.

When it comes to weight loss, most people focus on exercise and diet. They attend the gym for hours a day or start a restrictive diet that they usually end up quitting.

Independent eating is a much safer route to take and has shown to be more effective than traditional approaches for long-term weight loss. With independent eating, you're no longer tied to specific meal times and food groups. You can consume at any time you want, as many as you desire, and eat whatever you want! It's not an uncomplicated technique to master, but if done correctly it can help you lose more weight faster.

What Is Independent Eating?

Independent eating is when the individual chooses when and how much they're going to eat. The individual is responsible for how much they consume, and that's why it's called independent! At the end of each day, the individual writes down what they've eaten and drinks.

A common question is whether or not you're allowed to go out to eat, drink alcohol or eat snacks. The answer is yes! As long as you constantly check on everything you put into your body, there's no reason why you can't enjoy a few social drinks or dine at your favorite restaurants.

The main reason why people fail with independent eating is that they don't know how many calories, protein, and fiber they should be consuming. Independent eating for weight loss only works if you know the type of food you should eat.

Another common problem is getting an accurate picture of your diet. Independent eating is a commitment to the long term, so you can't just realize that you're not meeting your goals one week and quit. It takes months to lose weight with independent eating, so you must stick with it when the going gets tough.

There is no specific time that you should follow independent eating, but most people will start out by keeping track for 21 days. You can also try out tracking for 4 weeks or a month without taking any measurements at all. The goal is to get a general understanding of your diet habits.

When you track your food consumption, you need to ensure that you know what type of food you're eating. There are many different methods to determine the type of food, but the most accurate way is by using an app called Nutri-Score 7 (iOS) or 1 (Android).

Nutri-Score uses color coding for each food group. Green for protein, Yellow for fat, and Red for carbs. The idea is that the greener you place on your plate, the healthier you'll be eating for long-term weight loss.

It's an easy way to change your diet because you can use a plate or bowl and fill it with what foods you want. If you use a bowl, then mix everything before eating. If you use a plate, then divide the food up into four portions (protein, carb, fat, and fiber).

In the past, individuals did not feed as frequently as they do today, which is why we often get into trouble by eating too much and becoming overweight. However, eating too much is only one aspect of what makes us unhealthy—the types of foods we choose to consume are also significant contributors.

Western society has become so accustomed to processed foods that we no longer realize what these foods are doing to us because they are simply a part of our lives. We take them for granted and believe that they are good for us when in fact, they are harmful to our bodies. While there is definitely nothing inappropriate with indulging in a snack or meal from time to time, these products are practically the opposite of nutritious. If you find yourself snacking on junk food regularly, or otherwise consuming too many processed foods, you need to start making better choices, you have to be independent enough in order to take control.

CHAPTER 18:

Find Your Silent Mind

Silent mind dieting is the practice of balancing your intake and exercise habits to maintain a healthy weight without actually reducing calories. The calorie restriction associated with other diets is typically too difficult for people to constantly adhere to if they are not sure what they are doing, especially over the long term. This type of dieting can increase your chances of losing weight by increasing your awareness of what you need to cut out and what types of foods you should be adding back into your diet. A common misconception about diets is that you need to suffer to lose weight. A silent mind dieter believes that if you are suffering, then you are not winning. So, if you want your diet to be successful, then it should not represent a source of suffering for you. Embrace these changes over time and eventually, they will feel less like a diet and more like a new way of living.

A silent mind dieter is an individual who learns how to live by his/her own rules regarding food intake. They do not constantly consider the number of calories they intake at meals and only focus on eating when they are hungry. No special dieting techniques are applied and the individual is not being made to feel bad about what he/she eats. The main idea behind a silent mind diet is to bring awareness to the process of eating. This type of dieting can help you make healthier choices when you eat to lose weight and keep it off. The key to a silent mind diet is learning how to focus your attention on the moment of eating. This type of dieting can be very difficult for people who are always thinking about something else, whether it be work or school, trying to lose weight, or anything else. Instead of concentrating on eating the person focuses on his/her own breathing as they chew their food.

Eating while you are distracted puts your body in a state of stress and can cause weight gain as well as other health problems such as high cholesterol and high blood pressure. The amount of control you have when you are focused on eating is much less than when you are not. If you can make your mind still as to what is going on around you, your body will automatically put certain hormones into the bloodstream that will help suppress hunger. As soon as the stress caused by eating disappears, it causes an increase in appetite and weight gain. The secret is to know how to rid of food thoughts as soon as they come in and instead focus on something else. For example, instead of focusing on how many calories you are eating, you could think about what actions you have to execute to complete your tasks. You can even make it fun by thinking about anything from the outside world or what is going on in your life that would make it more interesting. Try not to focus on all the bad things that happen around you, and instead experience something fun or exciting that will help you lose weight.

The easiest way to become a silent mind dieter is by learning how to quiet your mind. Begin by focusing on your breathing. Try to bring all of your attention and energy to the fact that you are breathing. Once you have mastered how to concentrate on breathing, you will have mastered how to silence your thoughts. With adequate practice, it will become second nature and only take a small amount of effort for you not to be distracted when eating. The ability to quiet your mind and simultaneously eat will allow you to control how many calories you intake by focusing on what you are eating instead of what the food is. You will no longer have to think about how much exercise it would take to burn off all this food because it will just make itself simple by what goes into your mouth.

Once you become a silent mind dieter, it is best not to change anything else about what you are doing. If you are cutting out bread from your diet but decide to add a small amount of cheese to it, do not eat the cheese. You are attempting to stop a bad habit by replacing it with a less harmful one. If you try this, then you will begin thinking about how much fat is in that amount of cheese and that will once more divert your attention away from eating. It is best to avoid this because it will cause you to return back to the original habit.

To become a silent mind dieter, you must learn how to put your attention on yourself rather than what you are eating. For this dieting technique to work, you must focus on what you want instead of what you do not want. The more familiar you are with these thoughts, the less attention they will capture your conscious attention. There does not need to be a logical reason for it either. If you like cheese, then eat it. It is not something that you have to justify with being healthy. You can make it a goal to try and eat less cheese and some healthier alternatives every day if you choose to do so. You are no longer buying the food because of its calorie count or making yourself feel bad about what you are eating. It is now for your benefit so that you can lose weight and stay healthy. You will find that your body responds much better to the food you eat when you are in this frame of mind. You will find that if you want to cook some healthy food, it will taste much better as well, which will lead you to eat less.

The silent mind dieting technique is not for everyone. It requires great discipline and concentration to complete, and very few people can do it daily. It is suggested that you merge it with other types of dieting techniques to make it easier for yourself. The silent mind diet is only a small portion of a bigger dieting plan and should be used to provide a positive source of motivation.

One great way to incorporate the silent mind diet into your life is to find some successful pictures or posters. You can choose to put up pictures of yourself losing weight, or pictures of other people who have achieved great success. You could also simply use a beautiful image that appeals to you as a motivator.

Silent Mind for Dieting means incorporating mindfulness into your weight-loss journey. This can help you better develop healthy habits and break bad ones. It will also help you maintain a positive attitude—more important than weight loss itself—which is the first step to achieving success.

Mindfulness can help you to develop healthy habits that will stay with you for a lifetime. You'll also become aware of your bad habits, which will help you break them. It's not about restricting anything; it's about creating a balance that is beneficial for mind and body alike.

By incorporating mindful practices into your diet and lifestyle, you'll be able to reach your target weight while maintaining a positive attitude, which is the first step in achieving success.

Ask yourself: What is the point of having a six-pack if you're not happy with your body? It's pretty simple really. If you're not happy with the body you have, it doesn't matter whether or not you have six-pack abs. You will still feel terrible about yourself. It's all about changing your mindset before anything else.

"It's all about changing your mindset before everything else."

Changing your mindset is not just about losing weight. It's about improving your health and becoming the best you that you can be. It's about shifting your mindset, not just for weight loss but for a healthier lifestyle that will benefit you for years to come.

CHAPTER 19:

Free Your Mind and Don't Think Too Much About Problems

Clear Your Mind

Go through this day discreetly, doing fundamental breathing activities, and purposely relinquishing any burdens that may have been keeping you down lately.

You need a fresh start to draw in energizing new things. Here is a straightforward breathing activity to kick you off today.

Take a deep breath in through the nose. Fill your lungs and feel your stomach grow. Hold this for 4 seconds.

Discharge the breath through your mouth, similar to you is letting out a significant moan.

You're completely done! Rehash as regularly as you have to.

Make Space in Your Life

Look at your living spaces and clean up things that help you to remember negative considerations or bind you also firmly to the past (for instance, protests that help you to recall past connections).

Encircle yourself with things you partner with good faith, development, and enthusiasm.

Explore Your Goal

Consider what you trust you need. Presently ask yourself these inquiries...

- For what reason do you need it?
- Do you need it?
- When thinking about your objective, envision it showing in various ways until you get a feeling of the particular purpose, you're genuinely taking a stab at.

Put Your Goal Into the Words

Investigation with methods of stating what you need to show. Change the words around until you simply realize you've found the correct ones. Record them and put them up someplace you can see. One helpful method is to put them by or on your restroom reflect!

Make a Step-by-Step Plan

Note each progress you'll have to take to meet your definitive objective. This assists with guaranteeing you're progressing in the direction of something achievable and makes each stage concrete and genuine in your brain.

Create a Dream Board

This engaging activity just expects you to pick magazine patterns, photos, and words that best speak to the thing you need to pull in and join them such that you find moving. Be as imaginative as you like! For instance, if you are attempting to show your perfect partner, you may cover your fantasy board in pictures of sound connections, you know. You could likewise include statements of what you are searching for in an accomplice. You can utilize physical arrangement for this, for example, using photos and patterns as portrayed above or utilize online assets. Numerous individuals like to utilize locales like Pinterest as a type of fantasy board.

Pick a Manifestation Song

Discover a tune that catches all the sentiments you partner with your fantasy. For instance, you may pick a triumphant song of praise in case you're moving in the direction of a vocation or wellness objective, and a fantastic melody in case you're searching for adoration. Play it, move to it, sing it, and associate with it.

Basic Visualization

Put aside, in any event, ten minutes in a tranquil spot where you won't be upset and focus on building a maximally striking picture of the thing you need. Here are the absolute most helpful hints for improving your perception procedures:

- Envision not just the sight and sentiment of the thing you need to show yet, besides the various faculties. Picture the scents, sounds, and sensations as well.
- The utilization of reflection or hypnotherapy can likewise help dig further into your representation by shutting out interruptions and expanding your core interest.
- You can likewise utilize craftsmanship, composing, and music for perception! Draw, paint, or write your vision. Centerfold girl your work in a generally noticeable region, so you are helped to remember it regularly. Submerge yourself in this procedure, permitting yourself to feel it as if it's going on. It before long will be!

Design Your Affirmations

Utilize the expression (or expressions) to assemble attestations that fortify your conviction that you can draw in what you need. Let's assume them into the mirror, grin, and let them resound. You'll likely get the best outcomes on the off chance that you state them consistently. For instance, attempt a portion of the accompanying positive everyday certifications:

"I acknowledge my capacity."

- "All aspects of my life are copious and filling."
- "Each experience I have is ideal for my development."
- "I merit adoring. There is love surrounding me."

Write About Your Dream

Let your psyche meander unfiltered, and record as much as possible about your fantasy. For instance:

- What it resembles
- Why you need it
- How it'll be to live it
- Try not to blue pencil yourself by any stretch of the imagination, regardless of whether you get negative musings or emotions sneaking in

Uncover Negative Thinking Patterns

Check whether you can spot regions where constraining convictions and suspicions may hold you down and gaze them in the face. It is astounding what the number of our contemplations is subliminally negative!

Take a stab at asking yourself the accompanying inquiries...

- What are your uncertainty and tensions?
- How "reasonable" are your presumptions?
- What messages did you get when you were youthful that may lead you to figure you can't show your wants? At the point when you figure out how to respond to these inquiries, you can begin to reveal why you have explicit reasoning examples you do and how to recognize and battle whenever you get yourself on edge.

Challenge Negative Thinking Patterns

For each constraining conviction, you found in the past exercise, record a clarification of why you hold it. At that point, compose another, positive reasoning that you need to use to supplant the negative old one. You can utilize these to structure new attestations or simply look at the definite rundown once every day.

Take Stock of the Value You Have

Take care of yourself and consider things that support your confidence. On the off chance that it helps, take a stab at checking ten things you love and incentive about yourself. You have the right to have all that you need!

Connect With an Object

Discover something that speaks to your objective, for example, a stone, a bit of gem, or an adornment. Practice a perception while holding the article; at that point, ensure that the thing remains with you for the rest of the 21 days. It will ground you and help you to remember your latent capacity.

Additionally, consider examining the various advantages of gem recuperating. A scope of different gems and stones can help center the Law of Attraction work and lift your appearance power.

Multi-Perspective Visualization

Add another layer to your perceptions by envisioning your fantasy from an outsider's point of view. Notice new subtleties, develop a much increasingly amazing and energizing picture of what you'll accomplish.

Start a Gratitude Journal

Record 3–5 things that cause you to feel appreciative every day or every week, contingent upon your way of life. The reason for this errand is to fill you with vigorous positive imperativeness that causes you to vibrate at a high recurrence and improves your capacity to draw in progressively positive things to you. On the off chance that this is hard, make sure to consider what you underestimate every day. Things may not stand apart as something to be thankful for yet envision your existence without specific things.

Revisit Your Plan

Come back to the arrangement you made and consider where you are. Does anything have to change? Alter as vital and be satisfied with the means you've taken.

Look for Signs

The Universe regularly conveys signs to direct you towards the things you need; however, to see those signs, you have to get to your instinct. Today, keep your eyes stripped for rehashing expressions, incidents, or shock solicitations. These sorts of things may help you on your way. (P.S. Make sure to likewise pay a one-of-a-kind psyche to these seven great karma signs and otherworldly change manifestations!)

Give Love

Commit the day to consideration, empathy, and liberality, causing companions and outsiders the same to feel great. This, similar to your appreciation diary, encourages you to vibrate on a recurrence of wealth as opposed to one of need, placing you in the perfect space to show what you need.

Decide like you will have an accomplice, investigate excursions like you'll have the cash to pay for them, or buy garments like you'll fit into them how you need. This limits the vibrational hole among you and the thing you need.

Release What You Desire

At last, you have to figure out how to consider them to be in life all things considered, and acknowledge that the Universe will send what you need precisely when you need it. Put stock in your capacity to show yet discharge your longing and have a sense of security in the information you can and will have the life of your dream.

CHAPTER 20:

Develop Your Imagination

Dieting is a constant struggle for many people because they are never satisfied with the results achieved. This can be associated with a myriad of factors, but one of the most important is probably the mental barrier that we put up. Dieting is a physical activity and our body will always react in an attempt to save itself. The problem is that our mind reacts as well, often creating a vicious circle.

The power of imagination is great and it can help us to prepare for a diet or to cheat on one. For example, imagine how we will be when we finally achieve that perfect body that can motivate us to stick to the diet. On the other hand, when things go wrong, our imagination takes over and poisons our thoughts with doubt and feelings of failure.

To end this vicious course, we need to work on the mental aspect of dieting. We need to convince ourselves of our goals and to visualize the success. This is easier said than done, but it is possible.

The future is always a much brighter place than the present and that is what we need to focus on. Dieting does not happen in the present, it happens somewhere in the future when we will finally be rewarded with a great body that we deserve.

It may be difficult sometimes, but you have to keep working on your future. Visualize how you want to look, how you will feel when you finally achieve the body that you desire... This will make all the difference.

Think of dieting not as a struggle but as a challenge that you will overcome. Focus on the end result and try to focus on your progress towards it instead of the obstacles and setbacks that could occur.

Visualization is one of the best instruments for weight loss, but it is too often forgotten or confused with mere wishful thinking and dreaming. Visualizing your goals will help you achieve them. It works best if you do it as often as possible and especially when things get hard. Because it really is hard at times, but by helping yourself with mental reinforcement, you will overcome the challenges that dieting throws at you. Keep your head high and remember the reward.

Most people have tried to visualize their goals at least a couple of times in their lives. They probably spend a lot of time visualizing a desired future event. For the general public, visualization is a process where they picture their future within their mind. However, visualization can be used for much more than just that. It is a type of inner transformation that leads to seeing actual results in reality. A visualization is also a form of creative thinking where people can shape their lives using a specific purpose within their minds. The best part about the image is that a person may have envisioned that it doesn't have to rely upon the outer world's external events. It can depend entirely on a person's imagination.

There will be a moment when you will look back and see the progress that you have made. It is truly amazing how far you can go if you put your mind to it and know that you will never give up. Some people use visualization to help them achieve goals in all aspects of life, so why should dieting be any different? In addition, it is viable that visualization alone may help some of us lose weight faster than we could otherwise.

So, get to work on your mind and start visualizing your success. You will be surprised by what you can achieve.

Visualization for Creating a Plan of Action

It is normal to become stressed out or feel overwhelmed when trying to achieve new goals. For this reason, creating a plan of action using visualization can help you relax and motivate you to act. This technique is very effective if you use it before you go to bed to start planning the next day. You can also utilize this technique at any period during the day when you have 10 minutes of free time.

Below are three simple steps on how to do this:

1. Calm yourself down and make sure you are feeling relaxed. Sit down as it will help you get some rest from whatever you were doing before.
2. Close your eyes and start to visualize which things specifically that you want to accomplish for tomorrow.
3. Now, visualize those actions that you'd like to do in as much detail as you can and then ask yourself these questions below:
   - How would I like to feel?
   - How may I act around others?
   - Which specific actions do I want to take?
   - What do I want?
   - Which challenges may I face?
   - How can I deal with these challenges?
   - What results do I want to come from this?

The reality here is that people cannot predict all the things that might happen to them. When events happen unexpectedly, they can often ruin any plans that have been put in place. However, good planning isn't about planning around all possible obstacles, but it is more about adapting to the obstacles that life gives you. When you keep this in mind, you must affirm with yourself at the end of your session with "this or something better will come my way." By giving yourself affirmation, you are keeping your mind open to endless possibilities. This practice will result in more ready and okay with adjusting when unexpected things happen to you.

This process is not a foolproof plan. However, this visualization will help you envision possible situations that might happen. These scenarios will help you choose more ideal options for yourself as you continue to work towards your goals.

Visualization for Achieving Goals That You Have Set Out for Yourself

This visualization technique is the most important one when it comes to strengthening self-discipline. Using the visualization technique for setting goals brings a lot of value, but this technique does come with one major drawback. The most popular form of visualization is goal setting. Most people have used visualization about their goals at one time or another. However, this technique may not have worked for them due to one critical flaw. This flaw is that when people visualize their goals, they only focus on visualizing their end goal and nothing in between. They see within their mind's a big and flashy awesome goal that's going to be rainbows and butterflies. Yes, they are experiencing this using all of their senses, but they simply open their eyes after the visualization, feeling very inspired. However, this type of motivation is extremely short-lived because the next time this person faces an obstacle, it immediately deflates their motivation.

When this happens, people feel imagine the same goal all over again to create extra motivation. Though, because nothing happens after visualizing again, their motivation does not grow either. In fact, every time a person hits an obstacle and tries the process of visualization again, their motivation becomes weaker every time, and they start to lose more and more energy.

The mistake that these people are making is that they are not properly visualizing their goals. They only see the destination, but they don't understand that achieving a goal takes much more than just that. Achieving a goal is part of a journey that is full of emotional highs and lows, wins and losses, a journey of ups and downs. Due to this, these are the things that a person would also need to include in their visualization.

When a person visualizes their end goal, it is very effective in creating that desire and hunger. However, the proper way to use visualization is to spend 10 percent of your time visualizing the end goal and spending the rest of the visualization time thinking about how you will achieve your goals and overcome challenges. In some ways, it's similar to the form of visualization planning that we just tackled.

A person's end goal helps keep inspiration running in the long term, but it is the journey that helps a person stay motivated in the short term. To maximize the time spent on achieving small goals to get to your end goal, you must visualize those as well.

WEIGHT-LOSS PSYCHOLOGY FOR WOMEN

Below are five steps that you can follow to achieve this visualization:

1. Get yourself to a quiet place and sit down and close your eyes. Start to visualize the final stage of your goals. Imagine that you are experiencing and living the new reality that achieving your goal will bring you, using each of your five senses.

2. Slowly take steps backward from the end goal by visualizing the steps that you would take to achieve your end goal. Imagine the problems you might need to overcome; imagine yourself overcoming them. Picture yourself finding solutions to those problems. Continue visualizing until you reach the moment you are currently living.

3. Next, fast-forward from this moment and imagine which actions helped you overcome your problems.

4. After you finish this visualization, spend a few moments sending your future self some positive vibes and wish them luck on their journey.

5. When you exit the visualization, emotionally detach from the outcome of your goal. One factor that could potentially inhibit you is to have an emotional tie to a particular outcome. Alternatively, try to remain open-minded, flexible, and receptive to whatever is to come on your journey.

You can use visualization using those steps on a daily or weekly basis. Weekly sessions can be as long as 30 minutes, and you can keep your daily sessions shorter, so they are between 5–10 minutes. However, be sure that you are using your daily sessions to visualize the next steps on your journey to achieving the goals over the upcoming week. Doing this helps a person to continue making progress towards reaching their goal. After that, you can use your weekly visualizations using the five steps above.

The Benefits of Visualization

Here is something that not many people know: Visualizing an action or a skill before actually performing it is nearly as effective as physically doing it. Scientific studies found evidence of people's thoughts creating the exact same patterns of activity in their mind as it does with the physical movements of the action. When somebody is mentally rehearsing or practicing something in their mind using the visualization process, it impacts the many cognitive processes within a person's brain, including planning, motor control, memory, and attention perception. In layman's terms, the way a person's brain is stimulated when they visualize an action is the same as when they are performing it physically. Therefore, scientists can safely assume that the act of visualization provides just as much value as physically performing a task.

CHAPTER 21:

Eliminate the Superfluous

O f course, the problem with dieting boils down to one key issue: it's not an easy thing to do. There are just so many frustrating hurdles in your path that you rarely get to visible results. Your number one plan of approach is to eliminate the superfluous in dieting so you can see more progress with less effort.

To begin with, let's examine what superfluous is in dieting. Like I said earlier, the problem with most diets is that they have many restrictions and many rules that just add up to unnecessary frustration when you don't see results in a reasonable amount of time. There are many more diet rules than there are hard-earned or even noticeable results from following the rules. If you're like most Americans, then at some point in your life you've eaten food that no one needs. You read the label, checked the calories, and then ate it anyway. But let's say that it wasn't just a bad decision or an oversight on your part. What if every time you ate something that was no more than excess fat and sugar clogging up your system?

This is what happens when people eat superfluous foods.

The reason that superfluous eating is not as much of a problem in underdeveloped countries is that they consume nutrient-dense foods. They need to eat as many of these types of foods to survive, thus making it impossible for them to eat too many unhealthy ones.

Superfluous eating doesn't only refer to eating unhealthily just for the sake of tasty food. It also encompasses the people who stop exercising because they believe that their high caloric intake balances out any potential weight gain caused by exercising.

Another example is the person who eats so much healthy food, that they leave little room for anything else. If they do eat something like a piece of cake or a cookie, they feel like it's "bad" and have to punish themselves by either not eating again to make up for it or exercising excessively because of the caloric intake.

If you feel that you are doing this with your diet, then it's time to change the way you think about your food.

Superfluous eating is a difficult problem to fight simply because it's so ingrained into our society. The food world would have you manipulated that these foods are delicious and necessary. But are they really?

Superfluous eating can be overcome, but it requires a commitment from the individual. You have to be willing to educate yourself about the foods that you eat and learn to resist the temptation of superfluous eating. If you're like most people, then the hardest part will be breaking the habit.

The first step is awareness. You have to know what you're eating and why you are eating it. If you find yourself going for chips and salsa for dinner, then look at your reason for doing so. If it's because you just feel like it, then ask yourself why you feel that way.

You may be aware of what's in your food and not care about it or believe that it's not harming you, but this attitude is dangerous.

The foods that you are consuming are causing your body to worsen. They aren't giving you benefits and instead, they're causing damage. There are several ways that these foods can do this:

- The first of which is the number of calories these foods are containing. If you eat a giant burrito and it contains more calories than you should (especially if you're trying to lose weight), that's going to do some damage to your body. Not only that, but the high amount of fat and sugar is going to cause your blood sugar levels to increase too much which is just going to make it even harder for you to lose weight.

- Besides calories, the reason that your body does not produce an adequate number of hormones like leptin and insulin is that it's constantly exposed to excessive amounts of these foods. This causes your body to stop producing these hormones and the hormones that are being produced aren't doing their job effectively.

- Finally, eating unnecessary foods is going to cause you to gain weight. If you go out and eat a full meal of tacos, nachos, and ice cream then have to come home and do nothing but watch TV, then there's a good chance that your metabolism is going to slow down significantly for the rest of the day because your body was being stressed from consuming these foods. There are other concrete ways to eliminate the superfluous when dieting:

Seek Health, Not a Clothing Size

The idea of establishing an end goal brings up an important point for consideration. It can be very enticing to pursue a particular clothing size when you are in the process of losing weight. However, clothing size does not necessarily represent health or fitness.

Part of establishing renewed weight loss thinking is establishing new focused eating practices and then enabling your body to cope and change in retort to those modifications to your diet.

The problem with chasing a size is that many people set up size expectations that can only be achieved by strict deprivation dieting. Attaining a specific size may bring about a feeling of accomplishment in the short run, but these feelings will be short-lived if you can't maintain your new weight for the long haul. What's more, our body changes at different stages of our lives, which may necessitate a shift in sizing. Remember, no one sees the size on the tag but you! Yes, you are looking to transform something that no one else can see, but this inward transformation has little to do with your size at all. Instead of chasing a particular size, allow your body to respond naturally to your new eating habits. You will shed off weight and maintain it off if you establish focused eating habits. Seek physical and spiritual health, not a clothing size.

It Takes Patience to Grow a Fitness Habit

Habits take time to develop. Remember some of your most important habits, like brushing your teeth or recalling getting your bag or wallet with you no matter where you go. How did you develop those habits?

Most likely brushing your teeth was reinforced by a parent who routinely marched you to the bathroom and stood over your shoulder to make sure it was done. The purse habit, on the other hand, was probably reinforced by a terrifying "oops" moment when you rushed back to a food court table to discover your purse sitting unmolested where you left it... yep, I've been there.

I've heard it commonly repeated that it takes 3 weeks to develop a habit. When it comes to ingraining a habit, I wondered if 21 days was really enough for a habit to become second nature. Research in the European Journal of Social Psychology concluded that it actually takes an estimated sixty-six days for a person to pick up a new habit.

Over three months, the respondents decided on a new habit and communicated each time how instinctive the act is. After that specific period, researchers assessed the findings and discovered the estimated time it took for the respondents to develop a new habit was 66 days.

While their findings were centered on the time it takes to create a habit, we'll apply this to the time it takes to kick an old one and pick up a better one.

This number makes a lot of sense in light of my weight journey. As I mentioned before, the biggest defining factor for my successful weight loss, after years of failed yo-yo attempts, was the concerted effort to journal my thoughts and reactions to food for a full 50 days.

So, it's not surprising that this research study would conclude that it takes an estimated amount of sixty-six days for a newly discovered habit to become instinctive. At the same time, I also see some significance in the 3-week model because we often notice perceptible changes at this point. By three weeks, you will no longer notice that you are eating less food. Also, people are more encouraged to continue an activity once they receive the reward of noticeable feedback.

Factors for Developing a New Positive Weight Habit

If indeed it is going to take you just shy of ten weeks to successfully develop a new positive weight habit, it makes sense to consider some factors that will help ensure your success. To develop the two life habits, I mentioned earlier (teeth brushing and keeping up with a purse/wallet), habit formation required accountability and reinforcement, whether positive or negative.

Food Journaling as a Way to Analyze Yourself

Most people know that while in a food journal, they should keep careful track of everything they eat and drink so they can figure out what food combinations work best for them. The problem is that most people don't take the time to do it right. They either take pictures with their phone or rely on memory. However, if you're really serious about your diet, you might want to use a study technique called flash cards.

CHAPTER 22:

Lighten Your Home
From All That Has Now Passed

There's a lot more to weight loss than just restricting calories and exercising vigorously. Surrounding yourself with a healthy environment is the key to making it all work. When you're in the right environment, you have more of an opportunity for motivation and success.

It can be hard to identify what's holding you back from getting fit and keeping it off, but sometimes it might just be your home. "The place you live offers environmental cues that strongly shape your behavior," says Thomas Plante, a Ph.D., "You might have an excellent exercise program and a decent diet, but if your home is not conducive to healthy living, you won't be able to stay with your program."

Here are some simple tips to revamp your home for weight loss:

- **Make the kitchen an island of sanity.** If you've ever tried to cook a healthy meal in a cluttered kitchen, you know that the most suitable vicinity to be is in a clean kitchen, surrounded by only the things you need. "This isn't just about chopping vegetables," says Michael Fiutak, Ph.D. author of *The Research-Based Guide to Diet and Weight Loss*. "It's about eliminating distractions so that you keep your mind on what's going on in your kitchen. This is what is going to keep you from eating when you're not hungry."

- **Avoid a mall of mirrors.** Your bedroom should be for rest, not for showing off every inch of your body. "Being surrounded by full-length mirrors or even just reflective surfaces can promote a feeling of self-awareness and self-consciousness," says Plante. "You're more aware of yourself, and therefore more apt to judge yourself negatively. This can lead to eating in response to the anxiety that you feel."

- **Know what you're in for.** If you have a specific weight-loss goal, then make sure the rest of your house reflects this priority. Keep countertops free of temptations and clear surfaces off your walls so that if you see them, they won't trigger a desire for more food.

- **Make of sleep a sacred space.** Something as simple as scheduling your bedtime and making sure it's quiet can make a huge difference. "A quiet room offers plenty of places where you can get space from other people and focus on yourself," says Fiutak. "You have a better chance of staying with your program if you don't have to worry about what other people are doing."

- **Put plants in your house to benefit the health of your mind.** "If you have a cluttered home, then it's harder to tell yourself, 'This is not a problem,'" says Plante. "When we feel overwhelmed, we tend to surrender." The act of working on our minds is the best way to combat clutter and worry, and plants can help with this.

- **Read your food labels and drink in moderation.** Food labels can be loaded with sneaky words that set off cravings. For example, the word "butter" can cause you to want a high-fat treat, and the word "chocolate" can put you at risk for cravings. "If you're trying to lose weight, then be sure to read all the nutrition information on foods," says Plante. "Know what's in your food and your body."

- **Redecorate to distract yourself for short periods.** A new piece of furniture or a hand-painted wall can bring focus away from that cookie tray in the kitchen. "Just keep in mind that the best decorations are things that require some mental energy," says Fiutak. "For example, pretty pictures might not be effective because it's too easy to just look at them and get distracted."

- **Get your beauty sleep.** Studies show that sleep is the best way to boost your immune system. If you're not sleeping enough, it can be hard to stay on track with your eating plan. "Sleep deprivation has been linked to increased food intake and weight gain," says Fiutak. "This is because when we are sleep-deprived, we tend to eat more comfort foods."

- **Keep it clean by staying organized.** Appointment calendars, papers, and other clutter can make it difficult to keep your house in order, so keep everything in its place and have a place for everything. "Be sure to use the space where you store things wisely," says Fiutak. If you have several items scattered around your home, it will look like a junkyard.

Colorful fruits and vegetables can make a tasty and colorful addition to your countertop or table. "You might be surprised at how much fruit you eat when it has bright colors," says Fiutak. "The more color you have in your home, the less you'll think about making unhealthy choices."

- **Keep reminders out of sight.** If your home holds hidden temptations like a box of cookies or a stash of chocolate, then these things are likely to haunt your decisions about what you should and shouldn't eat. If you want to keep your eye on your goal weight, keep the reminders out of sight.

- **Break the cycle of emotional eating with a healthy home.** Being surrounded by healthy food choices can curb your appetite for junk food. "The more tempting foods that are available to you, the easier it is to give in," says Plante. "And if junk foods are available at home, then you are more likely to eat them instead of healthy choices. You can also make more nutritious choices by providing yourself with fresh fruits and vegetables in your kitchen.

- **Watch out for the urge to spend, spend, and spend!** Furniture, appliances, and decorations can add up quickly. It's simple to get overwhelmed with the idea to look for a brand-new design for your home but before you do so, think deeply first if it is a good investment. You don't want to buy impulsively and get the next shiny thing you see and then have a bad credit score when you get into debt."

- **Avoid processed foods.** A diet that includes too many processed foods can lead to excess weight, so avoid them if you want to lose weight. "Processed foods are heavily refined, stripped of nutrients, and contain synthetic additives, which make them a poor choice for weight loss," says Fiutak.

- **Don't forget about your fitness plan while trying to shed unwanted pounds.** "Fitness has a direct link to weight loss," says Plante. "When you're fit, you burn more calories and can eat more without gaining weight." Make sure that your fitness program includes exercise and healthy eating.

- **Stock up on fresh fruits and veggies.** A diet heavily reliant on fresh fruits and vegetables, whole grains, lean proteins, and healthy fats can help to keep you satisfied while keeping your waistline trim.

- **Make time for a healthy home-cooked meal.** Avoiding take-outs and eating foods at home is the most appropriate way to take control of your weight and keep track of your lifestyle. "If you cook yourself a nutritious meal, you're more likely to be satisfied and make healthier eating choices." Find ways to make cooking more pleasurable by slipping in some yoga exercises, meditating, or reading a book while you're preparing your dinner.

- **Get active with your family and friends during the holidays.** Many people who don't usually exercise will participate in seasonal activities like shopping, decorating, and visiting holiday displays. "Don't think of this as exercise," says Fiutak. "But if you add a little bit of activity to your daily routine, it will be easier to stay on track with weight-loss goals."

- **Beware of hidden calories.** Eating at home is generally healthier than eating out, but not always. "Hidden calories can add up quickly during the holidays," says Fiutak. "It's easy to overdo it when you're eating out on a busy schedule. The calories you don't burn off during the day are easier to consume at night."

- **Enjoy family traditions.** The holidays are a great time to gather together with friends and family (and eat some fantastic foods), but it's also an opportunity to create new traditions. Have everyone in the family walk a 5K or participate in a local holiday run. Make family fitness fun!

- **Strength-train.** It's easy to feel a little lazy during the holidays and skip the gym. However, skipping the gym is not going to allow you to meet your goals (and get fit) over the holidays. If you are doing strength training, just be sure that you increase your weight gradually throughout the holiday season.

- **Don't forget about health standards.** Each year, I like to set health standards for myself. This sets a goal for me and allows me to keep my fitness goals in check. For example, I like to make sure that I can:

- **Cut back on fat and calories when you do eat or drink.** It is important to remember that you are going to have a lot of times where you are going to be eating more food than usual during the holidays this year. And you must know how much food is going into your body. You don't want to be in situations where you are consuming a lot of calories that you can't use. So, if you are eating at a restaurant or someone's house, make sure that you eat slowly and try to limit portions.

- **Determine your portion control strategy.** You must select the appropriate strategy for your goals so it will work for you. Keep in mind your age, gender, weight, and activity levels when choosing a strategy.

- **Be sure you can afford a healthy diet.** You must choose to eat a healthy diet, but it is also important that you can afford it. Keep in mind your budget and how much money you have to spend on food. Make sure that you can still fit your goals into your budget so that you don't go over budget when trying to meet your weight-loss goals.

- **Make an exercise book a priority in your life.** It is important to keep exercising as part of your routine. Make sure that you are taking steps in the direction of exercise goals. If you aren't making time for exercise, then it is something that you will have to change. Don't be afraid to change your schedule around so that time for exercise is a priority in your life.
- **Read the nutrition labels.** You must study nutrition labels when shopping so that you can make healthy choices while still staying within your budget and eating on a budget.
- **Stock up on your favorite snacks.** You must have some healthy snacks on hand in case you're feeling hungry. If you don't have anything healthy to eat, then you might be tempted to eat something unhealthy. Be sure to make some healthy snacks for yourself so that you can control what goes into your body.

CHAPTER 23:

Enough Comparisons: Watching Others Makes You Fragile and Makes You Fat

How Do I Love My Body If There Is No Reason?

You stand and see yourself in the mirror and you are dissatisfied. Do you crave that your shape, your nose, your legs, your hair were like somebody else's? Why do we always compare ourselves? Why aren't we reconciled with our appearance? We have heard ad nauseam that we should love ourselves, despite our mistakes or flaws. This includes things related to our personality as well as our bodies. Nonetheless, there are very just so few individuals who can accept and be content with themselves. It is not about wanting to change. It is a commendable endeavor when one wants to achieve or retain their looks or care about looking more attractive.

At the same time, most people are much more critical, stricter with themselves than justified. They are continuously dissatisfied with themselves and don't see in the mirror what others see. Some girls feel a significant discomfort looking at each other, both because they don't like looking at each other in general, and because they don't like what they see. Where do these reactions come from?

What usually happens is that you don't look at yourself; you only see yourself concerning that ideal of beauty that you have in your head. This is where dissatisfaction creeps in. It has to do with the theory of social confrontation. We compare ourselves with those we consider better than ourselves; self-esteem is negatively affected. We all have a model in the head, a term of comparison that we have built by looking at years of magazines, advertising, and movies with perfect Hollywood princesses. The mantra must become one and only one: there is no need for me to compare myself to that model because everybody is a unique, generous specimen, rich in the indications of what I am.

Life would be much simpler and happier if we could accept ourselves as we are. A lot of negative emotions would be released, we would have less stress, and more of the things that really matter come into view. The bottom line is, if we need to change something, we can't do it until we make peace with the current state. This is a vicious circle.

The mind works, in effect, in a strange way. If we resist something, we get more of it.

After all, if we focus our attention on what is bad, we reinforce the bad. And what we pay the most attention to as we think about something will come true.

Everything that comes from you that relates to you is just yours: your feelings, your voice, your actions, your ears, your thighs, your hopes, and your fears. That's why you are unique. Be happy that you are different from anyone, that you look the way you do and that it is just you. Start to feel that it's your own body, not something separate that you need to live with.

Do you want your house to be just like anyone else's? Or do you love the little things that carry memories? Don't you love the atmosphere of your messy place after playing with your kids?

WEIGHT-LOSS PSYCHOLOGY FOR WOMEN

That's how you should feel about your body. You should understand that you don't need to compare it with anyone else's because it's impossible to compare unique things. Besides, who determines what beautiful and ugly mean? You should not compare your body to the celebrities' perfect-looking bodies.

You're not them. You are neither the next-door girl who, after three children, looks like she did at twenty, nor your friend who you think is gorgeous. You should not only accept your body, but you should fall in love with it. Do you think like Bonnie? Do you think no one could love you because you have some extra weight? Then ask yourself the following questions. Could you fall in love with someone only if they are perfect-looking? Would you really love someone because of their body? I'll go further.

Do we really love perfect-looking people? I bet you prefer your imperfect companion instead of a perfect-looking bodybuilder. You like the little faults of your wife, husband, kids, and friends because they belong to you too. We love imperfections better than perfections.

See? We don't measure people based on their weight. In addition, if you are happy with your body and your existence, it will also manifest in your radiance.

How Should You Love Your Body?

Imagine you have a fear of bugs that obsesses you. The psychologist might ask you to look closely at bugs until you get used to them, desensitizing yourself to the features that first terrified you. You can apply the same procedure to your body (Ferrer, 2015).

Here's an exercise that can help those who struggle to be happy about their imperfections. You have to stand in front of a large mirror and look at yourself as if you were doing it for the first time in your life, like never before, taking time for yourself. It must be a constructive and very careful observation. No distractions, no work commitments, no notification to pull your attention. Only you and the mirror. Next time you hate your body or any part of your body, stand in front of a mirror and look at yourself. Go from top to bottom and sort out your "mistakes." You will have to start looking at yourself from head to toe, objectively observing all the details, without comparisons or judgments.

Remember what that part of your body has done for you. When did it help, when did it protect you, when did it do something physically useful for you? Say thank you for something that was of help to you. Learn to practice gratitude.

Appreciate what you have and love your inner self. Don't let a scale or a size define your identity and skills. It is no use to criticize yourself fiercely when looking in the mirror.

Here are some ways to cultivate enormous gratitude in everyday life. When faced with a negative situation, do not be discouraged. Ask yourself instead what you can learn for the future and for reasons to feel grateful. Promise yourself not to be negative or not to criticize yourself for three days. If you make a mistake, forgive yourself and go on your way. This exercise will help you understand that negative thoughts are just a waste of energy. Every day, list the reasons why you feel grateful. The body is a miracle and you should celebrate all the gifts it has given you. Think about the goals you have passed, your relationships, and the activities you love it was your body that allowed you to do all this. Take note of it every day. Go to the next body part and do the same.

When you have reached your toes, return to your head again, to your face, and now, going downhill, just say to all your body parts, "I love you." Even if you feel a little stupid about it, don't stop. You see, you're going to have a completely different relationship with your appearance. And by the way, let's not forget, it's not a coincidence that it's called outer. What's inside is more important. But what's inside is visible outside. So, use your inner self to love your outer, and you will be much calmer, happier, more satisfied, and more confident.

Set the alarm and watch yourself for at least 40 minutes at a time. Doing so could change your life. Experts talk about the epidemic spread of body image disorder, a severe problem that leads us to see ourselves as inadequate every time we look at our bodies. According to research, 90.2% of women have an altered image of themselves and are not satisfied with their bodies, a fact that has a lot to do with how we look in the mirror. The mirror is your new weapon: from enemy to ally but learning to use it in the right way (Ferrer, 2015).

Compliment yourself. You should consider yourself and treat yourself with the same kindness and the same admiration that you would reserve for those you love. You probably wouldn't direct the same criticisms you do to yourself, to another person. Don't hesitate to compliment yourself, don't be too hard on yourself, and forgive yourself when you make a mistake. Get rid of the hatred you feel for yourself, replace it with greater understanding and appreciation. Look in the mirror and repeat: "I am attractive. I am sure of myself. I am fantastic!" Do it regularly and you'll begin to see yourself in a positive light. When you reach a goal, be proud. Look in the mirror and say, "Great job, I'm proud of myself."

Stay away from negativity. Avoid people who only talk badly about their bodies. You risk getting infected by their insecurities and dwelling on your faults. Life is too short and valuable to be consumed by hating yourself or looking for every little fault, especially when the perception you have of yourself tends to be much more critical than that of others. If a person starts to criticize their body, don't get involved in their negativity. Change the subject instead or leave. Wear comfortable clothes that reflect who you are. Everything you have in the wardrobe should enhance your body. Don't wear uncomfortable clothes just to impress others. Remember that those who accept themselves always look great. Wear clean, undamaged garments to dress the body the way you deserve. Buy matching briefs and bras, even though you are the only one to see them. You will remind your inner self that you are doing it exclusively for yourself.

Ask others what they love about you and what they consider your best qualities. This will help you develop yourself and remind you that your body has given you so much. You will probably be surprised to discover what others find beautiful about you; you have probably forgotten about them.

Surround yourself with people who love themselves. People absorb the attitudes and behaviors of the people around them. If your life is full of positive influences, you will also adopt them, and they will help you to love both your inner and outer. Look for optimistic people who work hard to achieve their goals and respect themselves.

Think of all the people who have reached important goals and whom you admire. They can be individuals you know personally or not. They are probably renowned and respected for the goals achieved regardless of the type of physique they have. Take the opportunity to remember that the body is not an obstacle to living or finding happiness. The body can help you pursue all your dreams and desires.

Think of your family, your closest friends, or a person you don't know personally but have always admired. Make a list of their best qualities. Then ask yourself if the image they have of themselves or their bodies has positively influenced their successes or prevented them from reaching a goal.

CHAPTER 24:

Stop Complaining and the Pounds Will Go Away

We've all been there. Maybe you're reacting to a comment from a friend or family member about your weight, or maybe you overheard a coworker talk about how much they love their latest meal while they were talking to someone else. Whatever the case may be, when we hear people talk about food and it makes us think about our own weight, we tend to get emotional. And being emotional, in turn, can lead us to say or do something that's not very productive for a healthier lifestyle. The main point is that complaining about your weight, talking about how fat you are, or how you wish you could eat whatever you want and not gain weight isn't helping you get any healthier. In fact, it may be doing just the opposite.

Consider this: If your goal is to lose some weight and be as healthy as possible, then constantly talking about how much weight you need to lose is counterproductive. When you do this, you're essentially focusing on that one thing that your goal is to get away from—eating too much and gaining weight. You're not visualizing how it would feel to fit into a nice pair of jeans, or how it would feel to be able to go for a walk without getting winded. Instead, you're probably just thinking about how badly you want food at the moment.

If you have a good support system of people around you who are trying to eat healthfully and get healthier, then it's probably not as important for you to focus on your weight.

You can get rid of those negative food thoughts: The more you hear yourself think negative things about your weight, the more you will start to follow it. "I wish I could still eat all of the pasta I want," you may think. "I wish I could live on junk food and never have to worry about getting fat." "I wish I never had to get up to exercise—that would make losing weight a whole lot easier." If you're feeling this way, then it's time to get rid of those negative thoughts. Remind yourself that you can still have some of those things that you like to eat, just not all of them and that you can still fit in exercise, and live a healthy lifestyle.

There are several approaches to get your health-related goals accomplished without focusing on weight loss or how fat you are.

Many people find that when they cut out things like sugar and bread, there are a lot of other foods they have to avoid. It's also a bit difficult for some people to accept in the beginning that this is a lifestyle change and not just dieting. So, we've compiled the top five reasons why you should try to stop complaining about your diet:

1. **Losing weight isn't just about what you can't eat, it's also about what you can eat.** If you love fresh fruit and vegetables, whole grains, and lean proteins like fish or chicken breast, you'll find that many of your favorite foods are actually allowed on a healthy eating plan.

The old saying that nuances are the spice of life is especially true when trying to lose weight. Because eating a wide range of foods helps keep your body in prime condition for burning fat instead of storing it. And if you think about it, it's this variety that can help prevent the dreaded diet-rebound effect. You may also find that you don't have to leave your favorite foods behind!

2. **Your mental health is bound up in losing weight.** A 2012 study from King's College London found a correlation between how fat a person was and the quality of their mood, as measured by their scores on the Hamilton Depression Rating Scale. (This study also showed that men with higher BMIs were more likely to be depressed.) Not only does being overweight affect your physical health, but it may also cause or worsen mental health issues like depression and anxiety.

3. **The longer you eat a "treat" food, the more you crave it.** And it doesn't matter if it's a piece of chocolate cake or soda pop that's making you fat. In fact, research suggests that it may not be the nutrient content of your diet that's at fault at all. It could be linked to something called "liking," which is about how much someone likes something they are about to eat, rather than what they are actually eating. If you eat food too often, you'll likely start to crave it and like it more, and that can make it harder to stop eating. One study found empirical evidence of this type of liking: It showed that rats would choose foods they had grown used to over new foods, even if the new foods were healthier for them.

4. **When you make peace with your diet, you'll feel better in general.** If you find yourself feeling better about your weight after you start losing the pounds, you'll likely feel better about your overall health more generally. And if that happens, you may even start to develop a new sense of confidence in your ability to make dieting work.

5. **Some people really do need to cut out fat from their diet.**

And you mustn't make the mistake of trying to go "completely" or "perfectly" vegan, vegetarian, low carbohydrate, or low-fat all the time.

It's more important that you make the choice to eat healthy foods, even if you find yourself occasionally eating some high-fat products.

But when you do have a piece of cake or a few slices of bacon, do something so that you can enjoy it without getting overly hungry or emotional later.

Or better yet, write down when and how you ate your treat and see what it is about that moment that causes you to feel regret.

At the same time, you can continue to try and lose weight and get healthier.

But if you're struggling, it might be a good idea to schedule a consultation with a registered dietitian or nutritionist just to make sure that your diet is balanced.

It can also be useful to talk about what's causing those weird feelings of guilt or shame when you eat.

You may be astonished at the number of individuals who end up being the complainer in groups. It's not because they are unhappy or down in the dumps, but instead because they are never satisfied with their current state of fitness.

The thing that so many people don't realize about this type of attitude is that it almost always backfires, and you end up feeling worse than when you started. If you tell someone that they are eating too much, or aren't doing enough exercise, you are just hurting their feelings and making them feel bad about themselves. If you complain about how much the person weighs, then you are making them feel like an outcast. The reason that people think it is okay to complain is that they don't want to take responsibility for their decisions.

Because of this, it will be very difficult for them to change their current lifestyle as a result of it.

If you want to help someone else, then let them know yourself. The best way to get others to change for the better is by example, and if you can do it in a way that doesn't make people feel bad about themselves then everyone will be more likely to want to change.

We all have days that are less than perfect. And while it can be cathartic to share your bad day with friends or family, there's a right way and a wrong way to do that. A recent study found that complaining may actually make you feel worse!

Solving the Problem

First, there's a big difference between complaining and venting. Venting is letting out your frustrations in a controlled way to help reduce their power over you. A complaint is something else entirely—when you complain, you're focusing on how things should be, not how to make them that way. When you complain, you're engaged in a negative feedback loop—one that doesn't lead to any solutions or changes.

When you complain, you're focusing on how things should be, not how to make them that way.

So how can you take the energy and emotions from a bad day and turn them into a positive outcome? Focus on what you can do to solve the problem instead of just being angry or sad about it. Think about what's getting in your way of fixing the problem and ask yourself if your attitude is helping things. In many cases, the frustration you feel is the very thing blocking your ability to solve the problem.

There's a lot of truth to that old saying "it's not what happens to you, it's how you react to it." When things aren't going your way, don't just complain about them! Instead, be constructive and focus on turning a bad situation into a better one.

Goal Setting

Goal setting is a powerful tool. It sets you up for success by aligning you to your desire while having a plan so you can take massive action in whatever ways make the most sense for you. So rather than complaining, act and set goals that empower you to go for it! It supports you in staying accountable to yourself. Goals are like that nagging best friend that won't let you off the hook when you tell them your biggest dream.

Goal Setting Ritual

1. Begin by writing out all of the desires you have for your body for at least 10 minutes. Don't overthink it. Just let yourself do a brain dump. Write everything that you desire no matter how confronting or silly it might feel.

Let yourself feel the release of moving all of that energy from your brain to the paper.

2. Now, recollect all of the desires you listed and pick the top three desires.

3. From those three, pick the number one top priority.

4. Write out what measurable goal can happen in the next 13 weeks. Make it as specific as possible. For example: releasing 1.5 pounds a week or jogging a twelve-minute mile.

5. Then write down all of the actions you need to take to reach that goal. Brain dumps here again.

6. Pick the top three actions that feel the most impactful and realistic for you at this moment.

7. Schedule those actions in your calendar and incorporate them into your life.

8. Continue to check in with your goals and actions every day to keep you inspired and motivated.

CHAPTER 25:

Couple Overweight: How to Deal With It

When obesity rates are up and normal-weight people are in an overwhelming minority, it can be easy to assume that the issue of overweight couples is just a positive side effect. That couldn't be further from the truth. Obese couples have more issues in their relationships than other couples, with more marital violence and infidelity among them. Even though these couples may not be able to lose weight on their own, they should still seek counseling so they can work through these issues together.

Once you've crossed the line and become obese, you're nearly three times more likely than normal-weight people to cheat on your partner. Even though partners in obese couples are usually aware of the extra pounds and sometimes try to make changes, it can be hard for them to succeed, and many will continue to have trust issues with their significant other. Being overweight can also lead to fighting over weight-related issues as well as infidelity. You may be surprised to know that women are more likely than men to be unfaithful, though researchers aren't sure why. What we do know is that these issues in overweight relationships can cause serious rifts. Obese couples are more likely to get divorced than normal-weight couples, and they also fight over weight-related issues more often.

If you're obese and your partner isn't, you should talk about how you can reach a goal of losing weight together. Just as you can't lose weight without support, you can't have a healthy relationship with your partner if you're unhappy with the way you look. Just because your partner isn't overweight doesn't mean that you won't argue about his or her eating habits, though. Healthy eating is important for both of you, and while many people on a diet try to ignore their partner's eating habits, this is one area where overfat spouses should be sensitive. Most people don't want to be in the vicinity of someone who's out of control around food. If one partner is constantly snacking or drinking sweetened beverages, he or she might be not only harming his or her health but also sending bad messages to your kids about the need for healthy eating.

If you're overweight, you can help your partner by taking on a healthier lifestyle yourself. You might not be able to make the decisions that your partner makes, but you can control what you eat and encourage him or her to do the same. There's no point in monitoring a spouse who continues to eat high-calorie foods, and you can't really offer support if you're eating more than your fair share of junk food. You may be amazed to discover that it's easier for your partner to follow a diet when an overfat spouse does it as well. She or he will be happier knowing that you're also trying to lose weight. If both of you avoid sugary drinks and high-calorie snacks, it will be easier for your partner to avoid these temptations as well.

Some obese people think that others would accept them more if they were partnered with someone who is also overweight. This is rarely the case, and if you end up in a relationship with someone who is also obese, you're likely to have even more weight-related issues than those who are overweight but date normal-weight people. You may get a ton of attention, but you'll also end up with even more issues in your relationship.

You'll want to talk about how you can work on your weight together so that you can be happier and healthier as a couple.

Many couples are shocked when they find out that their partner is overweight and don't know what to say or do next. You may feel like you're being left out of the relationship if your partner is obese, but there's no reason for you to stay silent if there are problems in your relationship. Question your partner to engage with you in a healthier lifestyle, and if you go on a diet, request that he or she do the same. Instead of letting your partner's weight make you feel self-conscious about your own body, use it as an opportunity to eat healthy foods and exercise regularly. You're more likely to stay with your partner if you're also committed to making important changes to improve your health together. Don't let your spouse's weight be a secret between the two of you.

If you're overweight, you should never be embarrassed about being obese. You won't be any less attractive, and if your partner is obese as well, he or she isn't going to lose any weight on his or her own. What you should do when dating someone who is overweight is trying to find out what caused the extra pounds. You may be astonished to see that your partner was overweight before you started dating, and maybe he or she is struggling to control his or her appetite because of a medical issue. While you should never settle for a partner who isn't healthy, you must try to aid your significant other to lose some pounds, if he or she isn't able to do it on his or her own.

If you're obese, find out what type of diet plan suits you best, and then try to stick with it. If you allow yourself to go back to your old eating habits, you're unlikely to be able to lose weight. Remember that when you're dating someone who's overweight, you'll need the same commitment to a healthy lifestyle as he or she does. If your partner is overweight and not following a diet, he or she might not be interested in losing weight, but it's still important for both of you that you lose weight if possible. Read up on healthy foods and how to eat smarter instead of snacking. Begin exercising at least three times a week, and make sure that your significant other begins doing the same. This is a great opportunity for you to both lose weight together and being overweight shouldn't keep you from having a meaningful relationship with your partner.

The problem with dieting is that it's tough when you have to convince your partner to go on a diet as well. The only thing worse than telling them they're fat and need to lose weight is convincing them of that.

First, go with their eating habits. If they do not eat out of home, do not invite yourself to their house to eat. Do your shopping at the supermarket, not at the grocery store. You will be amazed at how many calories you can save by eating in the privacy of your kitchen instead of giving them a piece of your birthday cake.

Next, you need to help them get rid of that bad habit of nibbling when there is food in front of them. You can do that by keeping a bowl of fresh fruit on the kitchen table. You can also introduce them to the benefits of chewing gum to avoid temptation.

Make sure that you don't use food as a reward for your partner when they do something good. Food is not a reward, and if they start to see it like that, it will be much harder to lose weight for both of you.

Don't constantly remind them about their weight problem and how fat they are. Everyone has their insecurities, and constant reminders will not help. Instead, focus on the positive changes that they've already made.

And finally, make sure that your fat spouse has a healthy social life outside of the house. Encourage them to spend as much time as possible with their friends and get them involved in activities that don't involve food at all. The last thing you want is for them to become depressed and start eating even more just because they are alone at home all the time.

Every year, more than two-thirds of adults in the U.S. are overweight or obese. More and more weighty partners mean an increase in health issues for both partners at the same time as well as a corresponding rise in obesity-related lawsuits. And yet, even while we know that obesity leads to negative health outcomes and that overweight and obese couples struggle with weight stigma at home, little research has examined how this can affect romantic relationships between spouses or significant others.

Most studies on weight stigma and coupling have centered on single people. Kathleen Cunningham, a professor at the University of Pittsburgh found that obese women in particular often face discrimination when it comes to partnering and mating. She noted, for example, that some researchers found evidence suggesting that obese women were less likely to be called or set up on dates than their average or overweight peers.

Through her research, Cunningham noted that couples in which one partner is overweight or obese may be at a higher risk of divorce; some research has suggested that this may be due to the weight bias couples face when dealing with health or weight issues.

Researchers from IZA and Western University found that although obese women in dating relationships were more likely than their average-sized peers to have been married before, they were less likely to report strong romantic relationships with their partners. According to the researchers, this may be because by making themselves infertile, obese women were more likely to leave their partners.

The researchers investigated whether obese men are also at a higher risk of divorce. They found that though some studies had suggested that non-obese men were more likely to get divorced than their average-sized peers, this was not generally the case; only a few studies on non-obese men gave statistics relevant to the issue of divorce.

Researchers at the University of Wisconsin-Madison found that as weight stigma increases, so does the likelihood that partners will break up. This may be because obese partners may feel that they have less of a chance to find a partner who is also looking for a relationship than their heavier counterparts.

A study by Teigen and Perry from the Department of Psychology at Iowa State University found that some couples with obese partners were unhappy with each other's weight, and this may cause them to split up. In particular, the researchers found that partners were more likely to break up if their obese partners had higher levels of body dissatisfaction or low self-esteem than their heavier peers.

On the other hand, some studies have also suggested that being married to an overweight or obese person can be beneficial for one's health. For example, a 2015 study found that weight loss among spouses was associated with a reduced risk of heart disease.

Cunningham cited some research suggesting that obese couples were happier than average-sized couples when it comes to romantic relationships, and this is associated with their higher value placed on body image.

CHAPTER 26:

Weight Stigma

Individuals usually see thin people and are impressed by their self-discipline, self-determination, or their willpower, and self-control.

Yet should it be considered great self-control or great willpower to avoid consuming foods, when you are actually not hungry.

It is true willpower or true self-control when you can avoid eating foods you do not notice at all and you do not get any reward rush out of it.

The plain truth is that anyone would be able to resist sugary sweets or any food under these specific circumstances, as there is no need for any willpower or great self-control to avoid foods when you are not actually hungry and when you have no rushes to worry about.

Even though thin people do not need any extra self-control or willpower in these cases, if they do need it, their self-control and willpower would function optimally since they are non-dieters.

On top of these extreme circumstances, dieters who need to struggle with dieting of any kind also disrupt their cognition which is especially effective over their executive function.

The executive function is a process that promotes and helps with self-control. Hence, people following strict dieting plans have less self-control and willpower in those situations when they need more willpower.

On the other hand, in the same situations during which dieters struggle, non-dieters have plenty of self-control and willpower even though they do not need it.

And there is also another fact if thin people were to eat delicious cakes, treats, and other tempting foods, their metabolism burns more calories by far when compared with the dieter's metabolism state.

All of this means that thin people are mistakenly given some credit for staying fit and in shape at this job that comes easier to them than for those individuals following some dieting plan.

These facts lead to the very cruel irony which makes it very hard to keep losing weight for individuals who have been following some dieting plan.

Yes, it is physically possible to lose weight in the long run, but just a small minority of dieters actually manage to keep losing weight for months or years.

Following the trend, this battle does not come without demoralization, stigma, and damages to their mindset which dieting does to their physiology both in the short run and in the long run.

No matter the obstacles and challenges, we have to work on changing the stigma surrounding weight, especially weight gain.

You are struggling with additional pounds does not make you weak in any way. The factors affecting weight gain and weight regain and have nothing do to with your dieting choices.

Hence, be impressed by every single step you take, be grateful for every small goal you reach, and remind yourself that you are not weak, but you are a victim of a very unfair battle.

This battle is won by only a few who are more focused on staying healthy than losing weight, who are determined to improve their weight not by any artificial means, but only in a natural way.

The Impact of Weight Stigma

The main question here is whether anti-obesity and anti-overweight attitudes are the ones contributing to these outcomes in obese and overweight individuals.

First, we need to clarify this term of weight stigma. It is stereotyping or discrimination towards individuals based on their weight. Weight stigma is also known as weight-based discrimination or weight bias.

One of the major health risks of weight stigma lies in the fact that it can lead to extremely increased body dissatisfaction which is one of the leading factors contributing to the development of various kinds of eating disorders.

When it comes to the best-known factor leading to the development of an eating disorder, it is definitely the very common and highly present idealization of being thin as seen in media as well as other socio-cultural environments.

However, it is never acceptable by any means to discriminate against someone based on any physical features and weight is one of them.

On the other hand, weight stigma which includes blaming, shaming, and concern trolling individuals who struggle with their weight, happens more commonly than we want to admit.

The fact is it happens everywhere, at home, at school, at work, and in some cases even at the doctor's office.

This tells us that weight discrimination is more prevalent than we think and according to the latest studies on the topic, it even occurs more often than age or gender discrimination.

Another truth is that weight stigma is very dangerous increasing the risk for different behavioral and psychological issues such as binge eating, poor body image, and depression.

In fact, weight stigma has been documented as one of the risks for low self-esteem, depression, and extreme body dissatisfaction.

Moreover, those individuals who struggle with weight stigma also tend to engage more often in binge eating.

They are also at a significantly increased risk for developing some type of eating disorder and they are more likely to be diagnosed with BED or binge eating disorder.

Those individuals struggling with weight stigma also generally report that their family members, friends, and their physicians are the most common sources of their weight stigma struggles.

When it comes to family members and friends, diet talk and weight-based teasing are more often than not related to extreme weight control patterns, unhealthy behaviors, and weight gain as well as binge eating.

This being said, weight stigma in health care is yet another very important concern showing the magnitude of this problem.

The topic which shows health care professionals and providers, when talking to overweight and obese patients tend to provide them with not valuable health information, tend to spend not enough time with them, and tend to see them as annoying, and undisciplined as well as uncompliant with their weight-loss treatment.

There is also a massive issue regarding popular obesity and overweight prevention campaigns. Attention is given to weight control and obesity definitely has skyrocketed in the past several years.

By doing so, the industry has ingrained words such as diet, obesity epidemic, and BMI into our regular vocabulary.

Unfortunately, since the rise of these obesity and weight control campaigns, weight stigma has increased by almost seventy percent.

These types of campaigns mean good and they are well-intentioned, by overemphasizing weight control and weight in general, they somehow encourage eating disorders providing counterproductive effects on society in general.

CHAPTER 27:

Reactivate Slimming Energy

Have you ever craved that you could have an awesome body just like most celebrities? If you think only celebrities can have it, you are completely mistaken.

Because we have a society today that gives so much importance and pride to beauty and includes achieving weight loss, you should not be wondering why people are into everything that promises a flat tummy. Celebrities are being adored not only because of their talents but also because of their sexy bodies. Aside from being perceived as beautiful, a flat tummy can also boost your energy as you tend to do more things and be more active if you flatten your belly and increase your energy.

Another good thing about weight loss and increasing your energy is it makes you more involved in your life. They say that we should live life to the fullest, and this is only possible if you can participate well in all areas of your life. With a flattened belly and increased energy, you will surely be more involved in your workplace, family and love life, and your community as well.

Boosting Your Metabolism for Weight Loss

Metabolism helps a lot in burning fat. Fat people are due to the reason that their metabolism is not burning at a faster rate. Metabolism helps to burn fat even once you are sleeping.

You can provide a boost to your metabolism; this enables you to consume calories at a quicker rate than before. A super lift to your digestion must be conceivable if you are not kidding. It is difficult, so ensure that you are happy to do it. You should invest a great deal of time and vitality to increase a super lift.

To achieve this, you would like to try the following things:

- **Spend around 40 minutes to an hour each morning and do a few activities like swimming, cycling, and running.** Attempt to do this in the first part of the day as it will be a lot more advantageous. Do this daily and make sure you follow it no matter what.

- **As an addition, spend 20 minutes within the evening doing equivalent exercises.** You can do it before or after dinner; it's up to you. Attempt an alternate exercise at once, this will keep you occupied, and you won't get exhausted.

- **Put intervals in your session.** Let's say 2–3 minutes after every 10 minutes of exercise. This will assist you in regaining your stamina and supplying you with some energy.

- **Build up your muscles with legitimate training.** This permits you to practice for a more drawn-out period and increases your metabolism. Divide muscle-building sessions on days and according to your body parts. Commit two or three days for a particular body part. Suppose Mondays and Fridays for your upper body, Tuesdays, and Saturdays for the lower body.

- **Make sure to have breakfast every day.** This provides your body with much-needed energy, and your metabolism will operate at an equivalent level. If you omit your mealtime then your metabolism will hamper, you ought to not allow this to happen and have meals a day.

- **Try to practice when you are in the market.** Park your vehicle away; this will make you stroll to the shop and will be an extra exercise for your body. In case you're inside the store, consistently make the strides, and quit utilizing lifts. Every one of these things offers you extra exercise and your digestion will go higher.

- **With a quicker pace of digestion, your body will consume fat a lot quicker.** Throughout the day it'll move, and even once you are resting your body will consume fat.

Remember that you should follow the above strides with consistency. Along these lines, you can have a decent eating regimen, great exercise, well-working digestion, and a very much-formed body. With this setup, it will involve time before you shed pounds.

Effective Ways to Increase Your Energy

It is prevalent to feel low energy at different times of the day. Many individuals experience what is referred to as the "afternoon slump." It is a feeling of low energy and sleepiness. It can definitely take away from the quality of your day.

The typical reaction is to succeed in for a few sugar products and caffeine. Although this is temporarily effective, it will lead to an even more fatigued feeling once your blood sugar levels begin to lower from the quick rise created from these foods. Some medical conditions can cause fatigue. It is vital to see your medical specialist and rule out any possible underlying medical issues for your low energy levels. There is a myriad of easy and effective ways to boost your energy levels.

Quality Breakfast

Breakfast truly is the most important meal of the day, especially if you want to maintain steady energy levels. There are specific foods that are very good choices for energy. Avoid sugary foods and simple carbohydrates such as white bread or white flour-based products. High fiber foods such as oatmeal are a great choice as it is filling and high in nutrient value. Proteins such as eggs, cheese, and lean cuts of turkey or beef bacon are foods that will provide you with energy.

Nutrient-dense foods are what help to increase energy. Instead of eating three large meals, having five mini-meals can be more helpful to a steady flow of energy throughout the day. This would include a late morning and a late afternoon snack as two of the mini-meals.

Good Snack Choices

Some great choices are organic nuts such as walnuts, almonds, and peanuts. They are very nutritious and are high in magnesium and folic acid, which helps to increase energy. For example, peanut butter on an apple or banana is energy-boosting.

Balanced Meals

The goal is to eat balanced meals that keep blood sugar levels stable throughout the day. You are looking for an ideal combination of lean protein, fruit, vegetables, healthy fats, and complex carbohydrates. Green vegetables like kale, broccoli, and collard greens are very healthy and nutrient-dense.

You can make it simple by making your snacks raw food choices. Normally, the raw food snacks would be freshly sliced vegetables such as celery, carrots, or fresh fruits. You can also add a helping of these raw foods to your other meals as well.

Stay Well Hydrated

Drinking enough amounts of water is very important. We are always losing fluids throughout the day through the natural processes of the human body. Most people don't drink enough water to replenish these lost fluids. You may not be able to drink the standard recommended 8 glasses per day, but you need to try to boost your fluid intake. An easy way to do this is to carry a water bottle with you to work and keep one in your car. Always have water handy. This will also prevent temptations of drinking unhealthy beverages such as sugary soda. Being well hydrated helps you to feel more energy and to fight fatigue.

Physical Activity

Getting regular exercise will boost your energy levels and help keep you healthy. Exercise increases oxygen levels in the blood. Try to exercise for 20–30 minutes daily. You can even break it up into 10-minute short intervals. You can take a brisk 10-minute walk or use a treadmill. There are many options. Simple effects like using the stairs as a substitute for the elevator can be a way to squeeze more exercise time in. You can also incorporate deep breathing techniques to increase oxygen levels. This will provide more oxygen to the brain, therefore, raising energy levels.

Exercise

Exercise 3–5 times per week. This is far and away from the simplest. Increasing your energy levels promotes overall health. If you would like to be a well-rounded individual with good mental and physical health, you should take exercise very seriously.

Don't Oversleep

Sleeping too much will cause you to be as drained as not resting enough, you just don't rest and your brain is not awake!

Complete all began tasks. If you begin something, finish it. Taking a gander at half-finished employment and knowing sooner or later you should have finished it will deplete you of vitality. Finish what you start!

Find something to get energized over-plan things to anticipate and get amped up for. We never have a concern rising right on time for something we are anticipating—customary timetable of occasions that we love, golf, motion pictures, fishing, anything. Excitement and enthusiasm are good for energy levels as exercise and diet.

Social Activities

The lifestyle choices you make can have a direct impact on your energy. If you live a life of late nights and inconsistent sleep, it will wreak havoc on your energy. Your social circle can rob your energy too. Being with negative people can eventually make you into a negative person as well. It's essential to try to create a social circle of friends who are positive and productive people. Having similar interests can be inspiring and helpful in your life. Family members that are draining on your emotions are another area of concern. Try to set limits and healthy boundaries to any negative relationships you may have in your life.

Conclusion

The loss of body weight is a common goal for many people. However, the amount of weight loss and how it is gained varies for women and men. For women to successfully lose weight, they must account for their added hormones, menstruation cycle, and emotional fluctuations to plan appropriately and maintain the desired change in body weight.

Some people have psychologically protectionist beliefs—such as "I can't be happy unless I'm significantly thinner"—that prevent them from losing weight. Other people who hold perfectionistic standards about their bodies (such as feeling fat if they have gained five pounds) tend to make weight loss harder by setting themselves up for failure.

These psychological patterns are often compounded by the media environment, which bombards people with an unrealistic beauty ideal and promotes weight loss as an all-consuming goal.

Weight-loss psychology is emerging as an area of study that explores this interplay between mindset, self-esteem, and body image. For example, some psychologists who specialize in this area help people develop healthier eating habits by looking at their relationship with food. Having to understand and learn the inner wirings of weight-loss psychology can help you achieve the weight goals of your dreams. Losing weight is not just about how you physically look. Rather, it is also about your emotional and mental well-being. When you are confident in yourself, when you have found a way to transform into the person that you want to become through losing weight, then that is the goal of losing off some pounds. You must remember that your happiness and health lie heavily on your shoulders.

Learning how to lose weight and reading about various tips and tricks is only the first step to reaching your goals. You must be able to apply it in real life so that you can see your endpoint. At times it may seem like everything is impossible, but you must acknowledge the fact that you are not alone in doing this. You cannot allow yourself to give up on your dreams just because of a few mishaps. Stand up and try and try again, no matter what.

This is not about body shaming people; it is about helping people get the body and the health that they want and deserve.

As women, we are often pressured by society to always look physically good, to have an hourglass figure, with a slim waist and wide hips. Nonetheless, you must keep in mind that their opinions do not matter and the only thing that matters is what you think and what you believe in. If you want to lose weight, you must make sure that you are doing it for yourself and yourself only. If you want to bring out the real you, you must look deep inside yourself without being bombarded by the words of those around you. Losing weight may not be a walk in the park, but when you eventually reach your goals, everything will be worth it.

Thank you for reading This book.
If you enjoyed it please visit the site where you
Purchased it and write a brief review. Your Feedback is
important to me and will help other readers decide whether
to read the book too.

Thank You
Keli Bay

Printed in Great Britain
by Amazon

68185997R00119